raising
healthy
kids

in an
unhealthy
world

DR. LINDA MINTLE

THOMAS NELSON
Since 1798

NASHVILLE   DALLAS   MEXICO CITY   RIO DE JANEIRO   BEIJING

Published in Nashville, Tennessee, by Thomas Nelson. Thomas Nelson is a registered trademark of Thomas Nelson, Inc.

Thomas Nelson, Inc. titles may be purchased in bulk for educational, business, fund-raising, or sales promotional use. For information, please e-mail SpecialMarkets@ThomasNelson.com.

Unless otherwise indicated, Scripture quotations in this volume are taken from the Holy Bible, New International Version (NIV). © 1973, 1978, 1984, by the International Bible Society. Used by permission of Zondervan. All rights reserved.

Other Scripture quotations are from:

The New King James Version (NKJV), © 1982 by Thomas Nelson, Inc. Used by permission. All rights reserved.

The Message (MSG), © 1993 by Eugene H. Peterson. Used by permission of NavPress Publishing Group.

This book is not intended to provide therapy, counseling, clinical advice, or treatment or to take the place of clinical advice and treatment from your personal physician or professional mental health provider. Readers are advised to consult their own qualified health-care physicians regarding mental health and medical issues. Neither the publisher nor the author takes any responsibility for any possible consequences from any treatment, action, or application of information in this book to the reader. Names, places, and identifying details have been changed to protect the privacy of individuals who may have similar experiences. The characters depicted here consist of composites of a number of people with similar issues, and the names and circumstances have been changed to protect their confidentiality. Any similarity between the names and stories of individuals described in this book to individuals known to readers is purely coincidental.

Formerly published as *Overweight Kids*.

Library of Congress Cataloging-in-Publication Data

Mintle, Linda.
    Raising healthy kids in an unhealthy world / Linda Mintle.
      p. cm.
    Includes bibliographical references and index.
    ISBN 978-1-5914-5283-6 (trade paper)
    ISBN 978-1-4016-0412-7 (repak)

    1. Obesity in children—Popular works. I. Title.
RJ399.C6M563 2008
618.92'398--dc22

                        2008009832

Printed in the United States of America
08 09 10 11 12 13 RRD 9 8 7 6 5 4 3 2 1

To overweight kids,
You are valued and loved for who you are, not for what you weigh.
May God's complete purposes be fulfilled in your lives.

To parents who desire to do everything possible to help their children
become all they were intended to be.

Acknowledgments

Writing a book on parenting overweight children is only possible after years of listening to families who experience firsthand the frustration and pain caused by weight issues. Many adults still feel the sting of teasing from those early years of being overweight. Others know how difficult it is to live in our culture of thinness and be overweight. Thank you for sharing your stories, your heartaches, and your triumphs.

Thanks to my children, Matt and Katie, and my husband, Norm, for once again freeing up time for me to write. Writing involves a sacrifice of time we all make together, and I appreciate your support, love, and help.

A big thank you to Joey Paul who allowed me to write on this topic, knowing it was a project I really wanted to do. To Laura Minchew who agreed that this was an important and timely topic we needed to tackle. I am thankful for your heart to help families and make a difference in the lives of children. To Marie Prys who so graciously accepted the job of editing with her very busy schedule and family. You are a gem!

Contents

Help Is on the Way

As a mother, I want the best for my kids. I will do just about anything to help them become the man and woman they were designed to be. However, in today's crazy world of diets and excess, it's no easy task to raise children who eat right and feel good about their bodies. But it can be done! We can raise healthy and fit children, and *Raising Healthy Kids in an Unhealthy World* will help you do just that.

As a licensed therapist in clinical practice, I have specialized for over twenty years in the treatment of adults, teens, and kids with weight issues. Our country is facing an epidemic of obesity as more than one-third of our kids struggle with their weight. As a parent, you play a vital role in keeping your kids from becoming another statistic of this growing national crisis.

We begin with a simple but important question: "How do I know if my child is overweight?" The good news is that the answer is easy to figure out . . . and having an overweight child doesn't mean he or she will stay that way. That being said, we don't want our kids to go on diets. We want them to stop gaining weight and grow into the weight they already have. And while the climbing obesity rates have to do with your child, family, and outside environmental forces, you can become part of the solution rather than the problem.

When you raise a child who is overweight, it's easy to feel like a bad parent or feel guilty for letting this happen. That kind of guilt isn't productive. So instead of blaming yourselves, let's focus our efforts on becoming informed and then decide what kind of life we want for our children and our families. No child has to be defeated by his or her size. There is hope. As a parent, you can establish an environment that encourages success. There are changes you can make that will make a difference. It's never too late to instill good eating habits in your children. In addition, the connection between body, mind, and spirit cannot be ignored. Our faith can empower us to move forward, to be transformed. As parents we shape our children's perspective for what they believe and how they esteem themselves and others—we are their earthly foundation.

There's an old saying, *Sticks and stones may break my bones, but words will never hurt me.* As adults, we know this isn't true—words pack a powerful punch. Our primary job is to help our children feel loved, accepted, and confident in life. With this nurturing, a healthy body image develops in our children, and they learn to find enjoyment and love through channels other than food. Please don't underestimate the power of our influence. Parents are the biggest motivators—both through their talk and their walk. While the focus of this book will be to help our children navigate this developmental journey, we must be acutely aware that our talk needs to be backed up by action in our own lives.

Our children are the greatest legacy we have. Their health and well-being are part of the chain that connects us. That being said, the battle of the bulge can be waged successfully as our children grow in confidence and look forward to long, healthy lives. Are you with me?

1

Is My Child Overweight?

Jack watched the soccer game and cheered for his eleven-year-old son. "Run, Michael! Come on, step it up," he yelled.

"Looks like he needs to run a lot more," the father next to him piped up.

"What are you saying?" Jack snapped back, feeling his anger rise.

"Just looks like your son is going a little soft on the conditioning, that's all," the other man countered. "He could run faster if he wasn't so chubby."

Jack kept his cool, but everything inside of him wanted to reach over and punch this guy out. Of course, that would be real mature! *Michael is chubby? How ridiculous! He just needs to grow a bit more.* But the soccer dad's comment lingered in Jack's mind. After the kids were in bed that evening, Jack asked his wife, "Do you think Michael is chubby? He did look bigger to me than the other kids."

"What?" his wife answered. "I don't know. I mean, he does have some baby fat, and he wears 'husky' pants, but I don't think of him as chubby. It's just baby fat. I'm sure he'll grow out of it." But Jack wasn't so sure. He began to notice Michael's eating habits were less than ideal and concluded that perhaps his son's weight was becoming problematic.

Though prompted by an insensitive soccer dad, Jack's concern is good. (Commenting on the weight of other people's kids is not recommended!)

Together, Jack and his wife need to decide if Michael has a weight problem—although without putting a premium on the comments of others. If his parents conclude that Michael is overweight, they will need a plan to help him grow into his current weight. Michael could be developing poor eating habits and ultimately be at risk for health issues in the future. Ignoring the problem or delaying action could make things worse in the long run.

The Signs

Our fast-paced lifestyles sometimes blind us to the fact that our children may be struggling with their weight. Such was the case with Jack in the story above. It took a third party to cause Jack concern over his son's weight and eating habits. A British study revealed that many parents fail to see their overweight children as overweight, and that kids themselves tend to underestimate their weight.[1] This may be due to the fact that the population as a whole has become heavier. When so many people have the problem, being overweight may seem like the normal weight. And because there is such a stigma attached to being overweight, parents and kids may deny the problem even if they see it. However, nothing changes when denial kicks in. Instead, we must acknowledge the problem and work to resolve it. The physical, emotional, and spiritual health of our kids is at stake. Parents *can* make a difference, but we need a plan.

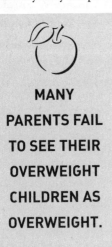

MANY PARENTS FAIL TO SEE THEIR OVERWEIGHT CHILDREN AS OVERWEIGHT.

The first step is to determine if your child is overweight. The easiest way to do this is to look at your child objectively and honestly. If your child looks overweight, he or she probably is. However, not all parents trust their own judgment when it comes to assessing weight issues. If you come from a family of overweight people, your judgment might be off a bit. If you were raised in a family of very thin people, you may see any extra weight as a problem. Or if you struggle with your own weight, you may feel you've lost perspective. If you have concerns about your child's weight, the family doctor or pediatrician is the right person to ask.

Keep in mind that some kids inherit a thicker or stockier body type, while others may be preparing for a growth spurt that requires them to temporarily up their calories. Babies and toddlers of a normal weight often have little potbellies and chubby bottoms, so these are not necessarily signs that a child is overweight.

Growth Charts

One way to evaluate your child's weight is to plot it on a growth chart. Growth charts are used by pediatricians to monitor a child's physical development. If you don't know where your child's weight falls on the growth chart, call your doctor's office and ask. Or the next time you go to the pediatrician, ask to see your child's growth chart. This information should be recorded at every doctor visit and placed in your child's medical chart.

Don't be afraid to ask for an explanation from the doctor or nurse—it's completely reasonable to ask them to explain the growth chart to you. The chart should show a growth curve with lines running through it. These lines are percentiles, a measure of the rank or position your child holds in relation to other children of the same age and height in the United States. These percentiles are used to assess a child's risk of being overweight. Generally speaking, a child who is at the 85th percentile or greater is at risk for being overweight or is overweight.

There are separate growth charts for boys and girls. In addition, one growth chart is for children between 0-36 months of age, and the second is for children between 2–20 years of age (see appendix A).[2] When a doctor tells you that your child's weight falls at the 70th percentile, this means that 30 percent of the children in the United States who are the same age as your child weigh more than your child, and 70 percent weigh the same or less. Likewise, if your child's weight fell in the 90th percentile, this means that only 10 percent of North American children the same age weigh more than your child. Thus your child weighs more than 90 percent of U.S. children.

So the percentile where your child's weight falls gives you an idea of whether or not you should be concerned about your child's weight. Any weight over the 85th percentile should be discussed with your pediatrician. Keep in mind that pediatricians look for trends over time when it comes to weight gain. A single number on a chart doesn't automatically mean your child has a weight problem. It's important to look at the overall growth pattern for your child and take into consideration the family's weight patterns as well.

Let's Try It!

Say your son is five years old and weighs fifty pounds. You would select the chart for boys (see appendix A) between the ages of 2 and 20 years old. Next, you would find the 5 (his age in years) at the bottom of the chart and draw your light vertical line. Then you would locate 50 (his weight in pounds) on the right side of the chart and draw your light horizontal line. At the point of intersection, you would place a dark dot. Following the curved line that is closest to that dot, we see that he is at the 95th percentile and is considered over-weight.

If you know your child's weight, you can plot it using the charts in appendix A. The first step is to choose the correct growth chart according to your child's gender and age. Using a pencil, locate your child's age at the bottom of the chart and make a light vertical line through that number. On the right hand side of the chart, find your child's weight (be careful to line up with the "pounds" column rather than "kilograms"!) and make a light horizontal line through that particular number. At the point where these two lines intersect, make a dark dot; then erase the light lines. The final step is to find the curved line that is closest to the dot—as you follow it to the right, you will find your child's percentile.

Body Mass Index (BMI)

A more accurate measure of body weight now included on pediatric growth charts is called the Body Mass Index (BMI). This measure represents the ratio of a child's weight in kilograms to the square of his or her height in meters. Hello, in English, please! In essence, BMI is used to determine whether a child's weight is appropriate for his height. To figure BMI, multiply your child's weight in pounds by the number 703. Next, divide that number by his height in inches. Finally, divide that number again by his height in inches. That number is then referenced on a chart we call the Body Mass Index to see what percentile the child falls into for his or her age group.

With children and teens, BMI is used as a screening tool to assess the scenarios of underweight, overweight, and at-risk for being overweight. The guidelines health care professionals use are as follows:

- A child is considered underweight with a BMI of less than the 5th percentile.

- A child is considered at risk for being overweight if his BMI falls between the 85th and 95th percentile.

- A child is considered overweight if his BMI is equal to or greater than the 95th percentile.[3]

One factor to keep in mind when figuring BMI is that some kids can score in the overweight range and not be obese. The reason is that BMI does not directly measure body fat. For instance, a very athletic child may have a large muscle mass and score in the overweight range yet not be overweight. It's important to talk to your pediatrician about your child's weight. That being said, most kids who score in the overweight range do so because of excess body fat rather than large muscle mass.

In terms of growth trends in kids, BMI decreases during the preschool years and then steadily increases into adulthood.[4] BMI is both gender and age specific. This is because boys and girls differ in their body fatness as

Let's Try It!

A ten-year-old girl weighs 71 pounds and is 55 inches tall. To find her BMI, you would perform these calculations:

1. 71 (weight in pounds) x 703 = 49,913

2. 49,913 ÷ 55 = 907.5

3. 907.5 ÷ 55 = 16.5

The next step would be to check the BMI chart for girls (ages 2-20 years) found in appendix B.[5] On the left side of the chart, we would locate 16.5 and draw a light horizontal line. Looking at the bottom of the chart, a vertical line would then be drawn through the number 10 (her age in years). At the point those two lines intersect, we would make a dot and then find the closest curved line delineating percentiles. The ten-year-old girl's BMI was 16.5—she currently falls at about the 50th percentile for weight, which means that half of all ten-year-old girls in the United States have a larger body mass index, and the other half (50 percent) have a smaller body mass index.

they mature, and body fatness changes over the years. It's important for your children to have a yearly checkup so that their growth and weight can be evaluated in order to establish trends and growth patterns. Physicians look for proportions that are constant. One single high number doesn't mean your child will be overweight for life or that you should panic. Instead, look for a growth pattern that indicates risk. By taking your son or daughter to the physician for a yearly wellness visit, your doctor can evaluate a child's growth more accurately in order to know how he or she is growing and whether you have reason to be concerned.

The Risks

When a child is overweight, parents should first make sure there is no underlying medical cause or condition. Witness the sensationalism of this headline reported in the BBC News: "Three-Year-Old Dies from Obesity." The subtitle reads, "Heart failure, caused by obesity, has killed a child aged three, it has been revealed."[6]

This story raised quite a stir and was touted as a wake-up call to all parents of overweight kids. Reading the headlines, you would think the parents stuffed their child with food, an act which then caused her to have a heart attack and die! Sadly, not all the facts were reported in the story. According to Dr. Sadaf Farooqi, one of the child's treating physicians, a genetic cause for the child's extreme weight gain was identified.[7] Her death wasn't caused by a heart attack that resulted from being obese. Can you imagine how those parents felt reading that headline? And that headline probably scared many other parents needlessly.

HEALTH RISKS INCREASE IN OVERWEIGHT KIDS.

The truth is that medical experts agree that dying from childhood obesity is not likely—other medical issues are usually involved. Drawing extreme conclusions about the health risks of childhood obesity is a bad idea. However, medical evidence proves children are healthier when they are at a good weight for their age and development. Scaring or blaming people will take us nowhere. The answer is to face the reality that health risks increase in overweight kids. As parents, we should want the best for our kids and do whatever is possible to eliminate these risks. Raising a healthy-weight child will help prevent long-term health problems.

Our own government estimates that 30 percent of the nation's kids are overweight or on their way to becoming so.[8] And the problem often persists into adulthood, placing more people at risk for disease.[9] According to Kenneth Land, professor of sociology at Duke University, obesity is a trend that is undermining our kids' health. Despite new medicines and advances in health care, Professor Land reports that there is an overall decline in children's health because of an increase in obesity.[10]

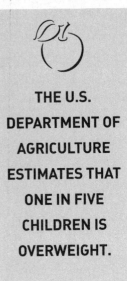

THE U.S. DEPARTMENT OF AGRICULTURE ESTIMATES THAT ONE IN FIVE CHILDREN IS OVERWEIGHT.

Doctors are very concerned as they witness increasing rates of child diabetes, cardiac problems, and hypertension. In fact, the Centers for Disease Control (CDC) reports that 60 percent of children between the ages of five and ten years old already have at least one risk factor for heart disease. And these factors also lead to other significant health problems.[11]

As a parent, you should be aware of the health risks associated with overweight kids. Children and adolescents who are overweight have higher rates of these medical conditions when compared to non-obese kids and teens.[12]

- Asthma. A link has been found between asthma and obesity with 77 percent of overweight children being more likely to have asthma than healthy-weight children.[13]

- Diabetes (type 2). The rate of this disease is more than 12.6 times higher in obese children. Cases of type 2 diabetes, the type that usually develops in adulthood, is now seen in overweight kids as well.

- Hypertension. This condition is nine times more frequent in obese children and is also a risk factor for heart disease and stroke. New guidelines now recommend that screenings for high blood pressure begin by age three. A new "prehypertensive" category for children whose blood pressure is somewhat elevated has been identified so physicians can recommend lifestyle changes in order to prevent full-blown hypertension.

- Orthopedic complications. This is due to problems of bowing and overgrowth of leg bones.

- Sleep apnea (the absence of breathing during sleep). This health problem affects 7 percent of obese kids.[14]

- Hyperlipidaemia (elevated levels of fat in the blood). This can lead to heart disease later in life.

- Constipation.[15]

A related health concern is one that often shows up in adolescent girls. It's called polycystic ovary syndrome (PCOS). This is a condition in which there is an accumulation of numerous cysts in the ovaries associated with high male hormone levels, irregular or absent periods, and other metabolic disturbances. Parents would typically notice excess weight, acne problems, and abnormal hair growth.

Obesity is related to this condition in that the distribution of fat seems to affect the severity of symptoms. The research on this condition shows a link to excess insulin, and obesity makes insulin resistance worse. Weight control and exercise help stabilize hormones and lower insulin levels.[16]

Whose Fault?

I couldn't believe the scene I witnessed at a fast-food restaurant one day. Honestly, I don't know what I would have done had it been me. A mom and daughter were having lunch . . . both were obese. A man walked past them and apparently decided it was his job to shame them into not eating (a strategy that doesn't work and is cruel). As he stood and watched mother and daughter consuming cheesy fries, Cokes, and double burgers, he commented on their meal selections. The mom was gracious and put up with the man's insults at first. She gave a forced smile and tried to ignore him.

But he didn't stop. "Lady, you're killing your kid, you know. It's one thing if *you* want to be fat, but look what you're doing to *her.* She's too young to know better." The atmosphere grew tense. The man was causing a scene. Again, the mom didn't say anything.

"Go on, keep eating," he goaded. Finally, she'd had enough. She took her child by the hand and tried to leave. Her daughter, who looked like she was about three years old, wouldn't move and was digging deeper into the cheesy fries, oblivious to the stranger's comments. With added force, the mom pulled her daughter away from the table and the two made their way out of the restaurant.

Across the aisle of the restaurant sat three preteen girls with their mom. They stared at the man who so rudely interrupted the other mother-daughter lunch. Then they laughed and went back to their meals. The three girls, who appeared to be between the ages of nine and twelve years of age, were downing the same fries, Cokes, and double burgers. The difference was that they weren't overweight. The stranger apparently felt no need to comment on their choices of food.

Many of us, if we are honest, want to blame someone when a problem emerges.

When people see an overweight child, they tend to blame the parents. Most people aren't as rude as the man in this story, even if they harbor the same thoughts or feelings inside. There is a false assumption that parents don't care about a child if she is overweight. Or worse, a conclusion is drawn that the parent is out of control. However, my professional experience with overweight kids and parents demonstrates that nothing could be farther from the truth when it comes to this assumption.

Overweight adults know they are overweight. The obese mom in the previous story probably felt like a failure and may indeed have given up. Most likely, she was a compulsive overeater and needed help as much as her daughter. Perhaps she struggles with feeling failed, shamed, and out of control with food and emotions in her own life. After all, it's hard to take your child on a healthy eating journey when you haven't gone there yourself. However, shaming this mom in public was hardly going to motivate her to make positive changes. She didn't need more ridicule. She needed empathy, a new plan for better decision making, and a positive reason to be hopeful.

In some cases, kids are overweight because parents feed them fattening food. The mom at the fast food restaurant wasn't helping her daughter by teaching her bad eating habits so early in life. But we can't assume this is why the daughter was overweight, either. The bigger picture is usually more complicated and the result of multiple influences.

Furthermore, not every parent of an overweight child is overweight. And many families have one child who is overweight, rather than all of their children. So to assume that it is all the fault of the parents is a ridiculous notion. Everything from genetics to unsafe neighborhoods plays a role in the growing obesity epidemic. In fact, depending on whom you ask, you can find blame for overweight kids anywhere. Remember the lawsuit against McDonald's? Or the one against Oreo™ cookies because they contain trans fat? Or how about blaming TV, video games, schools, soft drinks, doctors who don't encourage breastfeeding, motorized scooters . . . well, the list could go on and on. We could even blame God for giving us so much abundance in the way of food and comfort!

We live in a culture where there is plenty of freedom for making choices concerning the way we live our lives. When it comes to our health, there are good choices and not-so-good choices. But *we* make the choices. The younger our children are, the more we make choices for them, which does in fact tie us to their growth. Our job then is to model healthy behavior and teach them to make good choices. But assigning blame doesn't do much good . . . for anyone. Instead, let's look at some common reasons for why kids are overweight and then work on solutions. Leave shame, guilt, and rejection behind—they won't move us forward. Let's work to inform ourselves and then become empowered to make good choices in order to help our kids.

If you are struggling with your own weight and feel it is hypocritical to feed your child differently in the hopes of helping him grow into his weight, it's not. Now would be a good time to get help to overcome your weight issues while working on establishing a healthy eating environment for your child and family. If you don't have a weight problem, hang on. We're going to look at all the influences that impact your child—and suggest positive changes that will benefit any family's lifestyle.

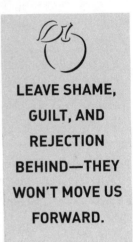

LEAVE SHAME, GUILT, AND REJECTION BEHIND—THEY WON'T MOVE US FORWARD.

The fact that you are reading this book is all the evidence necessary to see that you are concerned about your child and deeply love him or her very much. I applaud your willingness to do what's necessary to turn this problem around and help your child be healthy.

The Top Ten List

Overweight kids are the result of a number of factors, the least of which is uncaring parents. As we try to change these factors, it's easy to get frustrated, give up, and give in. So stay motivated, and when you feel like giving up, don't even go there. Little changes add up to big results in the long run!

The key to helping our kids is to identify the influences causing the most trouble and then make changes where necessary to help combat weight gain in those areas. For example, some parents will need to send a packed lunch to school rather than having their child buy a school lunch, while others will want to help their kids make time to exercise.

1. *Too many calorie-empty foods.* One of the most common reasons kids are overweight is that they have bad eating habits and take in more calories than they expend. When this happens, the excess energy from calories gets stored as fat. Parents are responsible for what and when their children eat, so we need to pay attention.

Our goal is to help our kids choose nutritious foods to encourage healthy growth and development. Children are responsible for eating the healthy food parents provide. "Empty-calorie" foods like sodas, chips, fries, and other high-fat foods that provide little nourishment need to be given special consideration, and perhaps taken out of the house entirely.

2. *Too little movement.* When kids aren't physically active, they can gain weight. If more energy is coming *in* rather than going *out,* weight gain is the result. This is perhaps the biggest factor as to why kids are more overweight now than in decades past. One of the biggest gifts we can give to our kids' health is to introduce them to a lifestyle that values exercise and movement. The reality is that kids live much more sedentary lives than they did years ago.

Remember When?

If I compare my own childhood to that of my children's, I see a big difference. As a child, I spent most of my afternoons and evenings outside running around the neighborhood playing games like kick-the-can, dodgeball, and other physically active games. I rarely watched TV. Furthermore, there were also chores to complete. The dishwasher was my brothers and me.

I don't remember having much homework until I was in high school. This meant that even during the school year, I was outside playing after sitting all day in a classroom. During school, we had multiple recesses and physical education every day. And as ancient as it sounds, I walked to and from school and rode my bike to my friend's house. I lived in a safe neighborhood that encouraged community play and physical activities.

3. *Genetics.* Though we would like to believe that we are overweight because of our genetic make-up, the truth is that genetics rarely *cause* overweight kids. They can increase a child's *risk* for being overweight, however. For example, if one parent is overweight, it's likely that half of the children will be overweight. And most of the children in a family will be overweight when both parents are overweight.[17] The tendency to be over-

Obesity Genes

One of the exciting areas of obesity research is aimed at trying to identify potential "obesity genes." New information is being discovered every day that may help us better understand the role of genetics in weight gain. In addition, researchers are trying to discover the role hormones and other body mechanisms play in terms of regulating appetite, hunger, and the sensation of feeling full.

One example cites a theory regarding the brain and hunger. About two to three hours after a meal is eaten, the stomach empties and secretes a hormone called gluetin. This hormone signals the brain and triggers appetite. You have the sensation of being hungry and want to eat again. You eat, gluetin levels drop, and your appetite decreases. When you eat, there are other hormones and molecules that tell your brain to stop eating. One of those is PYY. It acts in tandem with gluetin to tell you to be hungry or not be hungry. The hormone leptin also plays a role and signals your brain with the message that you've had enough fat and can stop eating so much.[18]

So what happens if someone's biology doesn't quite work in a helpful way and fails to turn off the "I'm full" feeling? Honestly, it isn't all clear to doctors how the genetics play into obesity. For example, researchers think that in some people leptin gets blocked and doesn't signal the brain like it should to tell the stomach it is full. Other researchers are looking at the possibility of viruses and infections causing people to overeat. And one Russian scientist is even looking at biological characteristics related to personality. He discovered that fidgety people burn more calories than those who are calm.[19] So who knows what will be discovered in the future?

weight can be inherited. This doesn't mean your child is doomed to be overweight if you or your spouse is overweight, but the risk will be greater. Good eating habits are a learned behavior, which means overweight parents may need to learn alongside their children.

That being said, genetic disorders can cause a child to be obese. A small proportion of children suffer from inherited chromosome-related disorders such as Prader Willi, Bardet-Bield, or Cohen syndrome. A child with Prader Willi syndrome usually develops an increased interest in food between the ages of one and four. This rare genetic disorder causes a child to be unable to feel full or control feelings of hunger. The result is excessive eating and an obsession with food, along with weight gain. When a child is born with Bardet-Bield Syndrome or Cohen Syndrome, childhood obesity is especially apparent in the trunk area of the body—it is in fact one of the defining features of these two syndromes. Bardet-Bield Syndrome also affects the vision. While all three of these disorders are rare, childhood obesity is a presenting symptom, and it is wise to have an obese child checked by a physician utilizing genetic testing.

When it comes to genetics, you get what you get. If your child is more at risk because of a family history of obesity, take special care to impact your child's eating in a positive way. Know the genetic risk, but don't let it determine your child's weight.

4. *Emotional eating.* One of the most common reasons we human beings are overweight is our tendency to eat because of our emotional needs. Whether it is because of their parents' marital tension or the threat of divorce, or to cope with being violated by sexual, physical, or emotional abuse, children eat to find comfort. Still others eat to cope with stress and anxiety over performance and perfection issues, or because of insecurities in peer relationships. When children feel rejected by friends, they can overeat. Eating can be a response to a multitude of emotions—including both positive and negative triggers.

In many families, food is associated with happy and celebratory times. In other families, food is used to escape or avoid emotional pain. For instance, when a child is abused, eating is one way to feel pleasure. Food doesn't talk back. It makes you feel good and requires nothing but your enjoyment. It also tends to be readily available. And like other

So Many Choices

Riding home from school in the car today, my daughter and I were talking about the new motorized scooters we have seen pop up in our neighborhood. They look like fun to ride but do not require any physical exertion by the person riding them. So we talked about the trade-off—do we want to go fast and enjoy the technology, or do we need to get more exercise by riding the standard scooter? Parents who buy the motorized scooters for their kids will need to make sure there are other ways for their children to get exercise during the day. (We opted for the non-motorized version.) Technology doesn't always mean improvement when it comes to the lifestyles of kids.

addictions, food can be used to numb out pain and life stress. That hot fudge sundae can be a sumptuous distraction from emotional pain, at least for the moment.

5. *Lifestyle and community changes.* Change is happening all the time. There are scientific advances, new technology, and a never-ending stream of "improvements" that contribute to being overweight. Community changes can affect children by causing them to move less and ultimately to burn fewer calories—parks are replaced with parking garages, there are no sidewalks for bikers, bus rides to school replace walking, etc. Over time, this lower level of activity adds up with unwanted pounds. A lifestyle change may be in order if you want to stay healthy and fit. Due to safety and wanting to protect kids, we often encourage them to play indoors rather than out. In low-income communities, access to healthy foods and markets is rare and can be expensive. If the meal deal at the local fast-food hangout is cheaper than a head of organic lettuce, a poor choice is made, though it is certainly understandable on one level. These realities require each of us to evaluate our living situations for the lifestyle changes that may be affecting our families negatively.

6. *Family patterns.* We hear so much about the face of the changing family—also whether or not these changes are good for kids. And in truth, when it comes to weight gain, many of the changes are not. Because kids have less time to spend with parents, since both Mom and Dad are working long hours, they tend to eat out of boredom and choose foods to comfort themselves. Many latchkey kids come home, sit in front of the TV, and eat. It's a way to relax from a stressful school day—adults often utilize this same practice as they seek comfort from the daily stresses of jobs.

Because of safety issues, latchkey kids are often told to stay in the house, which further encourages them to eat and sit. Another side of this topic has to do with the fact that more kids are in day care, which means parents can lose control over their child's fitness and eating. If your child spends significant time in a daycare, you may need to do some investigation and planning.

Lastly, the family meal is nothing more than a memory from a time past for many families. This tradition needs to be revived, and quick! Families on the run need to learn to preplan for their busy lives.

7. *The school scene.* Schools have become institutions where kids are less active while being exposed to more junk food and poor nutrition than ever before. You may be shocked to learn how commercialism has infiltrated our schools. Because of changes in educational policies, which often include dropping physical education requirements and program funding, schools are contributing to the poundage of our kids. Parents who want to combat the serious issues facing schools may decide to become advocates on the topics of health and nutrition.

8. *Advertisements and media.* The impact of advertisements and media on our kids is tremendous in terms of influencing what they eat. Never before have kids sat in front of so many screens and been exposed to so many negative messages from so many sources! Advertisements and marketing of food are big business . . . and kids make up a large segment of the market. Definitely our children influence the spending patterns in our families.

9. *A quick-fix mentality.* We are a pill-popping society with a desire for instant results. Dieting is big business in America, and the quick fix to being overweight is a promise many, many advertisers give while very few deliver. We've got to lose this mentality and realize that when it comes to improving our health, the correction doesn't happen overnight. Raising a healthy-weight child takes effort and intention on your part. Changes will need to be implemented over time with patience and persistence. There are no quick fixes, no magic diets, and no shortcuts. Only consistent changes that become part of a child's lifestyle will bring about slow and steady weight loss as children develop healthy bodies.

10. *Poor spiritual equipping.* Too many kids are fighting battles they are not equipped to fight. Whether it's the bully at school or the fudge brownies at the convenience store, kids really need adult guidance and intervention on how best to handle making choices. They need to be trained in how to overcome temptation and live right. And they need parents whose lives model overcoming their own weight-loss battles and victorious living. Many children need healing prayer for the hurts and wounds they have already experienced. Parents must equip their kids by living a vibrant spiritual life and teaching children a biblical worldview that can be applied to life's problems. The more secular our society becomes, the more we need children and adults who access the wisdom of God, are empowered by the Holy Spirit, and live transformed lives.

You Can Do It

If all of this seems overwhelming, it isn't. One step, another step, and then another step will eventually make a big difference. The results? Families who feel better physically, emotionally, and spiritually. Though there are certainly forces operating against good health, we have the power to overcome those and establish a healthy environment to raise a healthy weight child. So let's get started.

POINTS TO PONDER

1. Signs to watch for:

   - My child looks overweight.

   - My child's weight is at or above the 85th percentile on growth charts.

   - My child's weight is at or above the 85th percentile on BMI-for-age charts.

   - A health care professional has told me my child is either overweight or at risk.

2. Your child's health risks increase when he is overweight. Asthma, hypertension, and type 2 diabetes strike overweight children more than their healthy-weight peers.

3. Multiple influences cause kids to gain weight. It doesn't have to be overwhelming to help your child make a fresh start—instead, break down your lifestyle and see which segments need to be improved.

4. Analyze what areas you will need to consider making changes in order to help your child succeed in this battle of the bulge.

2
Let's Talk About It

Dear Dr. Linda,

My nine-year-old daughter threw me for a loop the other day. We were standing in my bathroom while I was putting on my makeup. The two of us were just talking, you know—about school, friends, music. Out of the blue, she asked, "Mom, am I fat?" How should I answer such a question, especially since she is overweight? I know her self-esteem is low and I didn't want to make things worse. But I didn't know what to say and also didn't want to lie to her. I could use your advice on this one.

—Tammy

Tammy isn't the only parent who has been faced with this question. Many parents have been in the hot seat over this issue! Understandably, Tammy wants to be truthful with her daughter, but also helpful. She knows her child's self-esteem is precarious at best. Hearing that she is overweight may very well cause the girl a great deal of hurt, and maybe even depression. So what is the best way to respond?

When it comes to weight, we need to be sensitive. The answers given for questions about appearance can have a positive or negative impact on a child's self-esteem. Translation: Stop a moment and carefully think about your answer before you respond! Having an answer prepared in advance is probably the safest route to take. And if this question has already come and gone and you said things you regret, it's not too late to influence your child in a positive way. I've spoken with many preteens and teens whose parents weren't so thoughtful about their responses. Girls with eating disorders often report their fathers called them "fat" or made degrading comments about their physical bodies. Even when the comments were made in fun, they hurt. Other kids talk about their mothers' preoccupations with thinness and the impact they had on their personal feelings about their bodies. When they heard Mom criticize her own thin body, these kids felt like they could never be thin enough.

THE ANSWERS GIVEN FOR QUESTIONS ABOUT APPEARANCE CAN HAVE A POSITIVE OR NEGATIVE IMPACT ON A CHILD'S SELF-ESTEEM.

When physical appearance and looking good at all costs are *over*emphasized in families, kids are at risk for eating disorders. And while parent comments don't *cause* an eating disorder, Mom's and Dad's little comments and behaviors *are* a factor, as we will see later. Be careful not to make disparaging remarks about your child's body. Statements such as those below can reduce a child's confidence and make him or her self-conscious.

- "You're getting a little chubby there."
- "Those fries are going to your thighs."
- "Your stomach jiggles like Jell-O.™"
- "Did you notice how fat that boy was?"

Avoid using nicknames that reference physical appearance. Names like "Tubbo," "Miss Piggy," and "Pudding Face" aren't funny, even if kids do laugh. Down deep, a child may question his worth or wonder if he is measuring up when called such names. Granted, some kids are less sensitive than others and can ignore name-calling; however, name-calling doesn't help any child feel better about himself.

There are times when you may have said something you thought was kind and gentle, yet your child misinterpreted what you said. For example, Tammy could say, "Honey, you do need to lose a little weight. You would probably feel better." Even though Tammy is saying this in love and trying to be gentle, her daughter might think, *My mom thinks I'm not good enough like I am. I have to please her by being thin.*

Though we can't control what our daughter or son thinks even when we speak with good intention, we must be aware of how sensitive a topic weight is for kids. It's so easy for our children to feel as if they aren't good enough because of their weight.

Refocus the Conversation

When kids ask questions about their weight, it's a good idea to gently move the conversation to a more general discussion about health. In other words, let's broaden the topic! Talk about your child's humor, thoughtfulness, kindness, or any other positive characteristic that comes to mind. Bring attention to achievements and character qualities. Discuss the fact that body weight and size are only two parts of a person's total make-up, while what is more important is her overall health and inner beauty. What you weigh is less important than being healthy, physically fit, and a person of good character.

The goal is to move the discussion away from societal expectations and instead gear the subject toward topics of health, nutrition, exercise, and character development. Let your child know that body size is not an indication of a person's overall health or worth. People with thin bodies may not be healthy, and not all people with big bodies are unhealthy. Talk about celebrities or pop culture icons your child may emulate. For example, Mary Kate and Ashley Olsen posters don the walls of many preteen girls. Mary Kate is very thin and was treated for an eating

What Should a Parent Say?

Like many parents, Tammy struggled with what she should say to her daughter when the question of weight came up. Here is one possible answer:

"What you weigh is only one part of who you are, and it is only important in terms of your health. What's more important is the kind of person you are and the way you make your friends feel special and included. I remember how you helped Michelle, the new girl in school, feel like a part of the group. Your kindness and care for her reflects an inner beauty much more important than the way you look on the outside. While it is important to take good care of your body, it is more important to love and serve others."

disorder. Let your child know that thinness doesn't mean happiness. Many Hollywood stars and other people starve their bodies in unhealthy ways in order to stay thin. Discuss unrealistic media images and explain that real people don't look like the airbrushed, computer-altered, perfectly lit images often seen on television, movies, and ads. Real people don't have perfect bodies. Our goal is to be healthy and live lives pleasing to God, not be perfect.

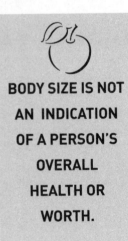

BODY SIZE IS NOT AN INDICATION OF A PERSON'S OVERALL HEALTH OR WORTH.

Behind the Question

If your child is overweight and you suspect he is eating for emotional reasons, it is necessary to get behind the question and to the heart of the matter. What is he thinking or feeling? Is something bothering him that he deals with by overeating? For example, a child might be shy. As a result, the child may be picked on by other kids and ultimately begin to overeat to comfort himself. Similarly, a girl who is physically developing may hear far too many sexual remarks and ultimately eat to deal with the anxiety she feels. Or there may be marital tension in the house that is so intense that your child escapes to his room and hides food under the bed to eat for comfort.

In these cases, rather than focus on weight, ask your child why he is asking about his weight right now. Is there something else on his mind? Is anything bothering him that he would like to talk about? Wait and see what he says. Allow your child time to share his concerns. Another issue may surface that is unrelated to weight that he or she is willing to talk about.

How About You?

Tammy needs to consider an additional question before she answers her daughter: how does she feel about her own body? If she dislikes her own body and feels fat, she will most likely send a negative message to her daughter. Girls between the ages of six and nine begin to worry about their weight—often because they have parents who are preoccupied with their own body images. Moms who talk about losing weight, complain about their thighs, or obsess over their abs in front of their children impact a child's self-image. Like the song says, "Oh be careful little mouth what you say!"

Be careful because children do listen to how you talk about your own body. What they hear you say about your body influences how they feel about theirs. When Tammy thought more about her feelings about her own body, she realized how often she made disparaging comments about her own body when standing in front of a mirror. What she didn't notice was that her daughter was listening. All moms are probably guilty of making negative comments about their bodies. I know I am! In the culture we live in, it's hard not to compare yourself to media images and come up short. But we as a culture need to realize that we are being fed a bunch of bologna when it comes to other sources defining our worth through physical appearance. We have to stop complaining about our weight, especially in front of our children, and accept the bodies we have while working on being healthy and fit.

We are created in God's image. People are the crowning glory of God's creation, yet often we forget this fact. When you look in the mirror, do you see a body that is wonderfully made by God? Or do you see flaws and focus on cellulite and sagging skin? Our culture glorifies youth and beauty over age and wrinkles. We listen to the influence of the media and let these messages seep into our heads about our own bodies to the point that the effects of the natural aging process our bodies go through are seen as ugly and unsightly. The bumpy ridges on our thighs are horrible. That double chin is all you see. And those wrinkles around your eyes and mine are *so* depressing, even though we can't stop them. Wrinkles and cellulite are a part of life.

> **WHEN YOU LOOK IN THE MIRROR, DO YOU SEE A BODY THAT IS WONDERFULLY MADE BY GOD?**

Friends, do you see how silly it is to focus on what our culture tells us? Should we really value nice skin and a perfect figure? Is that what God values? The Bible tells us, "The LORD does not look at the things man looks at. Man looks at the outward appearance, but the LORD looks at the heart" (1 Samuel 16:7). He wants us to care for our bodies, but the plan isn't for us to obsess over how we look. And often when we are overly concerned and vocal about our appearance, we forget that our children are watching and taking in our comments. *The way our children feel about their bodies is directly related to how we talk about ours.* The number of women I know who feel insecure about their physical bodies is staggering. No wonder our children are so insecure in this area!

If you have body image problems, you must address them in order to be a positive role model to your children. Make no mistake, your children will test you when it comes to this subject. I remember a time when my daughter was younger. I was toweling off from the shower when she walked into the bathroom. She looked at the cellulite on my legs and said, "Mom, that doesn't look too good. What is that crinkly stuff? Will I get that?" She looked genuinely worried, so I had to answer.

And I knew that what I said would make a difference in terms of what she thought about her own body. So I thought a minute and said, "Katie, this is cellulite, something women my age sometimes get when they get older. It's no big deal, just crinkly stuff. Most people have it. You might get it when you get older." I could tell she was still thinking about it. I was still missing something important in my answer, so I added, "And it doesn't hurt." A big smile came across her face. What a relief. Lots of people have it and it doesn't hurt! What more did a five-year-old need to know?

Countering a Negative Body Image

There are several strategies a parent can use to minimize the messages our culture gives in terms of body image. The first is to break idealized stereotypes, which means pointing out when culture is feeding us a line rather than reality. Counter the obvious lines—tell your daughter "thin" is not beautiful. Another important message to push: weight gain doesn't make a person bad or lazy. We want our children to learn that people are much more than their physical bodies—despite our culture's obsession with appearance. One of the reasons so many parents loved the movie *Shrek* was because the heroine and hero were not beautiful, thin people. Instead, the movie emphasized the other qualities of the characters. For once, the handsome prince didn't end up with the beautiful princess in a fairytale castle. Instead, two

> THE WAY OUR CHILDREN FEEL ABOUT THEIR BODIES IS DIRECTLY RELATED TO HOW WE TALK ABOUT OURS.

ogres fell in love with each other for the vibrant personalities beneath their green exteriors.

Another related strategy is to expose the lies of our culture. Perfect and thin bodies are supposed to bring success. It sounds silly, but certainly the message does get across: achieve the ideal body and then use it to your advantage. How often are the main characters on television shows overweight or unattractive? And what about all those commercials where people are having fun and selling products through advertising? It's rare to see someone who isn't beautiful or thin selling anything on television. Yet looking great is definitely not the only measure of success, or even the highest measure of our success as human beings.

Ask your child how she sees herself and reinforce a positive body image. Do the same when you consider your own body. Comments like, "Boy, I'd like to look like her!" tell your children you aren't happy with your body. And the reality is that looking gorgeous isn't the measure of a person, or what will ultimately bring happiness anyway. So make peace with your thighs. Love those sagging breasts that fed your babies! And please, let's avoid jokes about fat people. Parents must lead by example if they expect their children to follow.

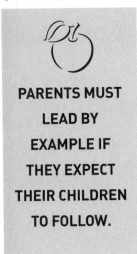

PARENTS MUST LEAD BY EXAMPLE IF THEY EXPECT THEIR CHILDREN TO FOLLOW.

In order to improve body image, search the Scriptures and read what God has to say about the gem of His creation (see appendix C for some clues). You will probably notice a disconnect between what God says and what our society says. The culture encourages us to compare and conform to images put before us in magazines, movies, and on TV. But God tells us to look deeper than the mirror for feedback. Ask God to share His thoughts and views about your body. As silly as it may sound, He will—through His written Word and through that still, small voice in prayer. God will speak to you if you listen, so ask Him to speak His truth to you.

Success Means . . .

What is the meaning of *success,* anyway? Webster's[1] gives the following definitions:

- degree or measure of succeeding

- favorable or desired outcome

- the attainment of wealth, favor, or eminence

- one that succeeds

Disappointed by this definition? I was. As a Christian, my success is not measured in such terms. Instead, the Christian would measure by the fruit born of a life lived for and sold to Christ.

Success is not defined by how many material things I own or whether I have memorable physical beauty. If it were, I probably would never own enough, and I would have to keep improving my looks since aging doesn't do much for our culture's picture of beauty. Happily, as a Christian I instead measure by these variables:

- how kind and forgiving I am to others

- how honest and authentically my life is lived

- to what extent I love my fellow man and God

The fruit of Christianity is peace, joy, and contentment—being pretty enough to grace a magazine cover for my looks or earthly achievements isn't to be expected . . . perhaps because even when one has those qualities, it isn't enough!

Proverbs tells us that "charm is deceptive, and beauty is fleeting" (31:30). Do you believe this? The verse goes on to say that "a woman who fears the LORD is to be praised." What a message to share with our daughters! But she'll have to hear this tidbit from you because she won't hear it much within the larger culture.

We can be free from negative body image when we realize and believe that we are accepted by God no matter what we weigh, secure because we are one of His, and significant because He created us for a specific purpose and destiny. God's love for us has nothing to do with how we look or what we do. And once we really accept and experience His love, it's hard to be negative.

Another point to cover is the fact that some weight gain is a normal part of growing and developing from a child into an adult. It helps to explain this reality early on so it is expected rather than feared. Overweight kids are encouraged to grow into their weight, but weight gain happens, especially around puberty. We cannot trust the media to educate our children when it comes to their concept of what is normal in regard to dieting and weight gain. And if a child has been overweight or is currently too heavy, they may fear *any* weight gain at all, even weight gain that would be considered healthy and part of normal growth and development.

Building Self-Esteem

Research tells us overweight children are five times more likely to describe their self-confidence as poor than kids who are average weight.[2] In therapy, many overweight children describe themselves as lonely, sad, and worried about a number of things, including their futures. As a result, they eat to cope with these bad feelings. Other overweight kids say they don't feel smart enough and that teachers don't understand them. In fact, there are certain psychological similarities between those who overeat and those who underachieve. Both groups often feel negative about school and classwork in general, having lost their academic confidence.

Overweight kids tend to believe that if they eat less and exercise more, *it won't make a difference.* Basically many feel they are stuck and cannot become thinner or healthier. They see the advantages physical beauty brings in our culture, yet feel they will never achieve it. But parents and teachers can help kids see that improvements can be made, that the situation isn't hopeless. The lessons begin early when it comes to instilling confidence and esteem in our children. The world tells children that self-esteem comes from the way they look, which products they own, how much they accomplish, and how well they compare to others. The reality is so different from these messages. We cannot rely on anyone else to teach our kids what the truth is. The best answer is to lead our children with a good example and consistently share a biblical view when it comes to questions of success and value. Genesis 1:26–27 tells us God made us in His image, both male and female. We are the reflected image of God Himself. The apostle Paul reminds us that those who don't know God are blinded to this fact. Because they don't have God's light (truth), they cannot see the glory of Christ, the very One whose image we reflect. Kids need to know the truth—they were created in God's image and reflect His glory. Second, kids need to know that when God created people, He declared His design good! We were His "good" idea! Our esteem comes from knowing our Creator and accepting His validation of us as good.

Yet this reality doesn't mean we are good. We are all sinners and fall short of God's glory, and only have been redeemed because of the sacrifice of God's Son, Jesus. As His children, God accepts and loves us just as we are. The more we know God and allow Him to work in us, the more He changes us from the inside out. We don't have to prove we are lovable, because God loves us in spite of our flaws and mistakes. It does little good to compare ourselves to others or judge by any cultural standards unless they line up with God's Word (which many of them don't).

The Bible tells us to treat our bodies with respect and take care of them because He made us and we have value to Him. He calls our bodies "holy temples" in His Word. One way to take care of our bodies is to eat right and exercise. Early on, teach your child to take care of her body, the holy temple where God lives. Finally, we must teach our children what God values—a heart that is true to Him and character that lives out biblical principles. When we do this, a healthy perspective will emerge that de-emphasizes the role of physical perfection and puts a premium on the development of godly character.

A Healthy Identity

Building a godly identity takes time and requires us to renew our minds on a daily basis. As parents we must listen to what children are telling themselves, talk to them about what they should believe, and correct their thinking when it comes to building an identity in Christ. Reading Scriptures that relate to a child's identity is a wonderful activity toward this end. Children need to know that God loves them, will never let them down, and is always dependable. This doesn't mean that bad things will never happen. But it does mean that when difficulty comes, God doesn't disappear. No matter what, God's presence is with us when we ask Him into our hearts. Ask your child if he has invited God to live in his heart. Kids need to understand that we can't earn God's love. We can only accept that love and bask in the identity we have in our Lord and Savior—new, beautiful creations!

Children's identities are strongly influenced by what their parents say about them. If their fathers are critical, demanding, or frequently tease them, children will typically feel inadequate and think God sees them the same way. This is also why so many adults are unsure about who they are—they still see themselves through the eyes of their parents rather than seeing themselves through God's eyes.

If you had loving, affirming parents, you'll have fewer problems accepting your true identity. But if your parents disappointed, hurt, abused, neglected, criticized, demanded, or violated you, and you felt you were never good enough to meet their standards, you have probably transferred these character qualities to God and are unsure of who you are. And the same is likely true for your children. They look to you to give them ideas about who God says they are. Affirm them; talk about their talents and gifts. A parent's life is a living testimony to his or her children and has great power when it comes to influencing body image, esteem, and identity, both physical and spiritual.

If you are alienated from God and unable to see yourself in His good esteem, you will have trouble conveying a different message to your children. And conversely, the more you are grounded in your own identity in Christ, the more likely you will equip your children to find their identity in the same source. We are so privileged to share this message with our children! Our children were designed to be family members, the daughters and sons of the most high God, and cherished by a Father who has only good things planned for those who serve Him.

"Jesus loves me, this I know . . . " Remember that song? Within that familiar hymn are the building blocks for godly esteem and confidence. Honestly answer the questions below. If you struggle believing these things, it will be difficult to authentically pass these beliefs to your children. Ask God to bring you new revelation of these simple but powerful truths so that you can in turn pass them on to your children.

"Jesus loves me, this I know." Do you know and believe this? Is this truth grounded deep in your heart so that no matter what, you know God loves you and His grace and mercy are yours?

"For the Bible tells me so." How often do you read the Bible as a guide to daily living and a source of revelation and parenting wisdom? Do you know the verses that speak to God's love, security, and acceptance? Can you quote them to your child and present them as foundational blocks for building esteem?

"Little ones to Him belong." Our children belong to God and He has a wonderful plan for each of their lives. We have to pray for our children, always seeking the will of God for our lives and theirs. Invite God into the process of building your child's identity and esteem.

"They are weak, but He is strong." When your child struggles or feels weak and hopeless, can you help him see that this is when God can be strong in him? Have you found this to be true in your own life, or have you turned away from God when life throws you a curve? Because of God's spirit in us, we can do all things. It isn't by our might or power but by His Spirit living in us. Can you testify to this truth in your own life?

From the top, let's make a few substitutions based on the idea that your child's perspective of God will be powerfully influenced by your parenting.

"Mom and Dad love me, this I know." Does your child know this? Have you made love conditional and based on how she looks, complies with the rules, performs in school, sports, or other activities?

"For Mom and Dad tell me so." Do you tell your child regularly that he is loved? Do you hug, kiss, and cuddle your son or daughter often? We all long to hear the words "I love you" with no strings attached, and we like to hear those words often.

"Little ones to Mom and Dad belong." Does your child feel a sense of belonging and attachment to you that is deep and secure? Is she secure in the knowledge that Mom and Dad will help no matter what, that her parents are on her side? Will Mom and Dad stay together and fight the battles of life?

"I am weak, but they are strong." I'm not equating parents with God, but it helps children to know that when they feel hopeless, teased, rejected, or down that Mom and Dad are there to bolster them up. Do you encourage and build up your child with praise? When stress is high and the pressure is on, are you strong because of the way God is working in you? Do you turn to God in your weakness, surrender to His love, and ask Him to work in difficulty on your behalf?

> A PARENT'S LIFE IS A LIVING TESTIMONY TO HIS OR HER CHILDREN WHEN IT COMES TO INFLUENCING BODY IMAGE, ESTEEM, AND IDENTITY, BOTH PHYSICAL AND SPIRITUAL.

We must believe that God is who He says He is, and that we are who God says we are. And we must convey those beliefs to our children in order to build a solid foundation that won't crumble.

God,

Raising a child in today's world is an awesome challenge and can't be done without depending on Your wisdom and guidance. Thank You for providing both through Your Word and prayer. Continue to help me as a parent to understand the depth and breadth of Your unconditional love. Give me revelation of how much You delight in me and accept me regardless of my physical appearance. When I feel weak and don't know what to say or do to help my children, give me Your thoughts and words. Allow my children to discover their true identity in You and to feel esteemed as Your children. May they feel totally secure in You and never question their worth, knowing the extravagance of Your sacrifice and love. Amen.

POINTS TO PONDER

1. Weight is a very sensitive topic for most children. How we respond to questions about weight matters in terms of how our children feel about themselves.

2. When questions come, steer the discussion away from weight and toward a broader concept of your child's health and character.

3. Strive to provide unconditional love and affection to your children, just as God loves us . . . no matter what.

4. One of the biggest gifts we can give our children is the gift of helping them find God and their identity in Christ, and ultimately, esteem.

3

Not a Lifelong Battle

Dear Dr. Linda,

I am the parent of an overweight child and I am worried. Everyone in my family is overweight and I don't see any hope for my daughter growing up any other way. I don't mean to be so negative, but I think I'm being realistic. No one in my family has conquered the weight battle. I thought about putting my daughter on a diet but then I know how many I have already failed and I don't want to do that to her. Should I send her to one of those weight camps?

If your child is overweight, you are not alone. Look at these statistics: Twenty percent of kids ages 2–5, and almost one-third of kids 6–19 years of age, are at risk or overweight. And if you are a Mexican-American or African-American kid, you have a four in ten chance of being at risk or overweight.1 These days, many children are putting on extra weight.

You may be wondering if your child's weight will be a lifelong battle since it has emerged at such a young age. Such thoughts can be very discouraging for parents as they long for the best for their kids. The good news is that dealing with weight doesn't have to be a lifelong struggle. Attacking weight issues early in life by establishing good eating habits and healthy lifestyles will help alleviate extra weight that might not be so easy to address later in life. Four rules make up the backbone of my plan to help your child grow into his or her weight.

Rule #1: No Diets

In order to avoid weight obsession and future weight problems, *do not put your child on a diet.* When a child is put on a diet, he could miss getting the nutrition he needs. Growing kids are still developing and need a well-rounded diet with many essential nutrients to grow strong and healthy bodies. Dieting often eliminates food groups and important nutritional components that kids need.

Furthermore, when kids are put on diets, research shows they are more likely to *overeat.* That's right—overeat! Many will sneak "forbidden" items and begin to develop an unhealthy relationship with food based on deprivation. The fact is, kids want what they can't have. In truth, I don't recommend dieting for adults either. When you diet, you have to deprive yourself of certain foods, and that deprivation just makes you want those items even more. Dieting is a setup for long-term failure.

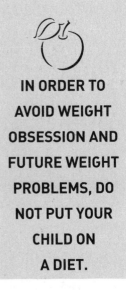

IN ORDER TO AVOID WEIGHT OBSESSION AND FUTURE WEIGHT PROBLEMS, DO NOT PUT YOUR CHILD ON A DIET.

Professional weight management programs do have a place—there are times when it is appropriate for a child to seek that type of treatment. However, these programs are reserved for children who are very obese and in need of extra help. We will look further into this option a little later in the book. For most parents, the goal will be to help your child stop gaining additional weight and instead grow into his current weight—a goal that will not be met through dieting.

Rule #2: Don't Become the Food Police

There are no bad foods, but our eating habits can be bad. So say dieticians the world over. Though it might be easier to label foods "good" and "bad" in order to maintain healthy eating habits, this is not the best way.

The reality is that no food has to be forbidden if it is eaten in moderation, which is the main goal of healthy eating. We don't automatically know which foods are healthy choices, what they do for our bodies, and why we should eat them—these are pieces of information we must learn. Children must be taught that foods bring various consequences in terms of how they make us feel and grow.

Many parents opt to become the food police instead of teaching their children to enjoy food with balance and moderation. They monitor their children, policing mealtimes and snacks to keep kids from getting into "bad" food. The problem is that becoming the food police creates power

Food Policing vs. Example Setting

Food police tend to require their kids to give a reckoning of all foods eaten over the course of the day, generally after the kids come home from school. But this action tends to make most kids resentful as well as secretive when they eat something on the "bad" list. A better approach would include focusing instead on good nutrition as it relates to a child's health. Talk about which foods give brain power and will help energize him at school. Then go over the school menu and talk about which foods encourage thinking and refueling the body. A good lead-in for such a conversation is, "We can feed our brains by choosing brain food [have him list what he thinks those may be], or we can feed our appetites by choosing foods that make us sleepy and inattentive [again, have him tell you which foods those might be]." Let him know the choice will be his.

Granted, kids don't always choose the healthy foods, but hey, neither do we! The important thing is kids learn to connect choices with consequences, and they learn that eating impacts their bodies. For example, we encourage drinking milk over soda because milk has calcium that builds strong bones. Sodas offer nothing in the way of nutrition. If kids want strong bones, which of those foods would be a better choice? Children will make good food choices with encouragement and support, most of the time. When they make a good choice, reinforce it with lots of praise.

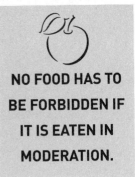

NO FOOD HAS TO BE FORBIDDEN IF IT IS EATEN IN MODERATION.

struggles between kids and parents over food, usually because parents feel that eating has gotten out of control (which certainly may be the case). And though their motive is good, this approach doesn't work. Policing food results in kids becoming secret eaters, because they don't stop craving those foods, even if the food is labeled as "bad." It actually makes them want the food even more and will only end up leading to more power struggles. The better path to take is to lead by example.

Rule #3: Make It a Family Affair

One of the most important things to keep in mind when helping your overweight child is that changes have to be made in the family, not just for the individual child. For parents, this shouldn't be too much of a sacrifice because we love our kids and want to provide them with the best possible lifestyle. Actually, it's not a sacrifice at all considering everyone will end up healthier!

What this means in practical terms is that you, your spouse, your teen, and anyone else who may live in your home will need to make some of the changes suggested in this book. It's not a good idea to single out your child to live differently because he or she has a "problem." Consider an overweight child instead as an indicator that changes need to be made in the family as a whole. Changes such as cutting down on fats and sugars, exercising more, reducing media time, and eating more nutritional foods in general are all good choices that will benefit everyone. Those family members who are already practicing good eating habits will serve as great role models.

Here's an example of what *not* to do. In the Smith home, only seven-year-old Jimmy is overweight. His older sister Tiffany is thin. Jimmy's parents are at healthy weights, mostly due to their physically active jobs.

Because only Jimmy had a weight problem, the family opted to have him work on the problem on his own. As a result, the Smith's household stock of junk food and soft drinks remained. Whenever Jimmy would reach for a snack from the chips and cookies in the pantry, his mother would say, "No, Jimmy. You can't have that food. There are some carrots in the refrigerator you can munch on." Meanwhile, Tiffany had free rein and regularly snacked on chips and soda in front of her brother. In the evenings, while the family enjoyed eating ice cream and cookies for dessert, Jimmy was offered a piece of fruit.

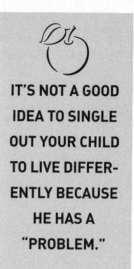

IT'S NOT A GOOD IDEA TO SINGLE OUT YOUR CHILD TO LIVE DIFFERENTLY BECAUSE HE HAS A "PROBLEM."

The result? Jimmy felt singled out and deprived, and it didn't seem to him that his family was trying to help him, even though that was their intention. Jimmy felt like he was abnormal and even bad since he was not given the same tasty foods as the rest of the family. The carrots and fruit were viewed as nothing more than punishments! Eventually he will want to sneak those tasty foods that are within the pantry, which will lead to power struggles and resentment.

A better plan would have been to modify the entire family's eating habits so that Jimmy didn't have to face this battle alone. Families have to be included in the treatment of weight loss in order for successful weight loss to be maintained. The reality is that good eating habits benefit everyone, whether one family member or all family members are overweight.

Perhaps this approach seems unfair. Why should everyone in the family modify their eating if only one person seems to be having a problem? The answer is easy—you are committing your family to a healthier lifestyle, which is hardly a punishment! Kids live and learn *in families*. They are highly influenced by their caretakers and give more attention to what parents do rather than what they say. Parents are role

Approaching the Subject

If you have some less-than-willing members of the family who are resistant to the changes you are trying to implement, consider using these lines to get your message out:

"We've all been eating too much junk food and not feeding our bodies good nutritional foods that help us grow, think, and function at our best. So, our family is going to begin making changes in the way we eat and exercise. Our first change is _____ [fill in the blank with one item you want to change]."

Thus the emphasis is not on the extra weight but on developing strong, healthy bodies. And since you are only implementing one change at a time instead of several, it should be easier to make your case heard to the other members of the family.

models, teachers, trainers, coaches. This can be a frightening thought, because we adults often have bad habits that may need changing, especially when it comes to eating and exercising. However, what a great motivator to know we are teachers! The healthier our lifestyles, the better chance we have of passing on good habits to our children. What a wonderful gift to give them . . . as well as helping ourselves in the process.

Take a moment and think about your own eating habits and weight. Ask yourself a few hard questions:

1. How do you feel about your body?

2. How do you talk about your body in front of your children?

3. When you evaluate your own eating and exercise habits, what kind of a model are you for your children? Can you improve your own habits?

Given today's fast-paced world and the stress of our lives, most families need to make a few adjustments in order to positively impact their overweight kids. The good news is that changing habits as a family builds support within the family. Parents and siblings can support each other by encouraging one another to make good choices. And the outcome for everyone is better living.

Rule #4: Set an Example of Moderation and Balance

In our culture, excess is more celebrated than ever before. Daily we are prodded to supersize, take that break we deserve, and have it our way. The message is that we should indulge in whatever feels good for the moment. Food is no exception.

The concept of overweight is about excess—excess fat from excess food. The goal of any healthy eating program is to eat in moderation. Another word for it would be *balance*. Through my work with teens struggling to overcome eating disorders, I have come up with the following explanation: When you eat too little and severely restrict food, it's called anorexia. When you eat too much, feel guilty, and throw it up or get rid of it, it's called bulimia. Both represent extremes in eating. The goal is to learn to eat moderately—to not restrict and not overindulge. A continuum of this principle would look like this:

Food Restriction - - - - - -➤**Moderate,** - - - - - -➤**Overeating**
                              Healthy Eating

Anorexia   Eating   Bulimia

Emotions often parallel this same continuum. Take the emotion of anger, for example:

Denying Anger - - - - - -➤ **Controlled** - - - - - -➤**Venting Anger**
                but Expressed Appropriately

Emotional Restriction   Hitting, Throwing,
                                               Name-calling, etc.
                                               (Emotional
                                               Bingeing)

The goal is to seek balance as we live. For example, if we feel anger, which is normal, we must acknowledge it, feel it, and deal with it in a healthy way. We want to avoid extremes and embrace moderation, especially when it comes to eating and food. If a child is given the option of eating as much candy as he wants, many will indulge until they are sick. Then the groans and moans can be heard. Too much of a good thing is too much! Even kids will concede that eating all the candy one wants ends in a tummy ache. So the lesson parents must teach is one of moderation. A sweet treat now and then is fine, but eating too much candy on a regular basis results in stomach aches in the short-term and probably a trip to the dentist in the long-term!

The same is true for other parts of kids' lives. Playing a video game for thirty minutes is a great way to have fun. Being glued to the screen for three hours is excess! And for studious kids, hours of studying must be balanced with physical activity and fun. This isn't generally a popular lesson; but since when is parenting about being popular?

With this rule it's absolutely a must that our lives reflect balance and moderation. Do we work too much, drink too often, spend impulsively, oversleep, shirk responsibility, compulsively overeat, or worry to death? Are our lives balanced in the areas that count? If not, it's hard to teach kids what we won't do ourselves . . . and don't think they won't notice the discrepancy. If you binge eat and overindulge at the fast-food counter by supersizing everything you eat, your kids will do the same. Take a look at your fast-food tray before you look at theirs.

What Do I Do?

If you are reading this and feel out of control in some areas of your life, please don't give up or walk away feeling condemned. Confess the problem to God. Then accept His grace and begin to make changes today. You don't have to "fix" everything at once. And you don't have to wait until you are "perfect" before you help your kids with balance and moderation in their lives. The important thing is to decide as a family to work on the trouble spots and try and bring more balance to life as a whole. The Holy Spirit will empower those who truly desire to make those changes.

As we surrender to God, He will help us. Friend, the fight with weight is not about willpower—it's about surrender. When we surrender our problem to God, we accept and own it. We confess our weakness and take responsibility for it where we can, and we allow God to empower and transform us. Take the first step and bring your sorrow before the God who made you and loves you.

And if you struggle with addictions, food problems, or other excesses, get into counseling and work on those issues. Take the lead and show your kids you are committed to a life of balance and moderation . . . for all of you! It's an act of courage to admit your own defeat, so there is no shame in this, only hope as you surrender the problem to God and ask for help.

Take the Quiz

Before we discuss eating habits, it's time to find out where you are when it comes to eating habits. You may want to take this quiz again in several months and compare your answers to see the improvements firsthand. Understand, there are no right or wrong answers here. By taking the first step of reading this book, you are working toward change. The next step to improving your eating habits is to see where your family is at, so honesty really counts! There isn't a key for answers here, or even a scale for winners and losers when it comes to eating habits. So why not take a few minutes to see where your family stands when it comes to eating habits?

What Are Our Eating Habits?

1. My family eats meals together
   a. every day
   b. several times a week
   c. rarely
   d. never
   Goal: Eat meals together every day

2. When we eat meals, the television is on in the background.
   a. yes
   b. no
   Goal: Television off during meals

3. My child eats in front of the television
   a. never
   b. rarely
   c. occasionally
   d. frequently
   Goal: Eat at the kitchen table

4. My child eats breakfast every day.
   a. yes
   b. no
   Goal: Eat breakfast daily for a good nutritional start to the day

5. When my child comes home from school, he or she eats snacks of
   a. fruit, cheese, protein, and other healthy foods
   b. chips and sodas
   c. sweets
   d. other _____
   Goal: Make provision for snacks such as those listed in (a)

6. In terms of the number of sodas my child consumes, he or she
   a. rarely has a soft drink
   b. has one or two during the week
   c. drinks them daily
   d. drinks more than one daily
   Goal: Rarely has a soft drink or is limited to one or two per week

7. My child eats at fast-food restaurants
   a. never
   b. rarely
   c. maybe once or twice a week
   d. several times a week
   Goal: Rarely or at most once a week—with improved food choices

8. When we go to fast-food restaurants, my child supersizes the meal
   a. never   c. occasionally
   b. rarely   d. frequently

   Goal: Never

9. My child sits in front of screens (television, video games, Internet, etc.)
   a. 0–2 hours a day   c. over 5 hours a day
   b. 2–5 hours a day

   Goal: 0–2 hours a day

10. Our family exercises together.
    a. true   b. false

    Goal: True

11. Our family believes we should finish all the food on our plates.
    a. yes   b. no

    Goal: Children should learn to stop eating when they are full

12. My child exercises
    a. less than 30 minutes a day   c. 60 or more minutes a day
    b. 30–60 minutes a day

    Goal: Exercise for 30–60 minutes a day

13. My child buys food from school vending machines
    a. never   c. occasionally
    b. rarely   d. frequently

    Goal: Never or rarely

14. My child's school lunch is healthy and nutritious.
    a. yes   b. no   c. I have no idea

    Goal: Make provision so your child can have healthy lunches

15. My child has daily physical education (PE) in school.
    a. yes   b. no

    *Goal: PE every day, even if you have to become a school advocate
    to make this happen*

16. My child's homework each night requires about
    a. 0–30 minutes   c. 1–2 hours
    b. 30 minutes to an hour   d. over 2 hours
              Goal: 30 minutes to an hour

17. People in our family eat when they are *not* hungry.
    a. true   b. false
        Goal: Eat because of physical hunger and not for emotional reasons

18. Mealtimes are relaxed and friendly in our home.
    a. never   c. occasionally
    b. rarely   d. most of the time
Goal: Avoid stress and chaos during meals and encourage a relaxed atmosphere

19. Our family eats at regular times
    a. never   c. sometimes
    b. rarely   d. most of the time
              Goal: Meals are scheduled

20. There are plenty of healthy foods for snacks and mealtimes in our home.
    a. yes   b. no.
        Goal: Have plenty of healthy snacks and meal foods on hand

21. My child is rewarded with special foods.
    a. yes   b. no
              Goal: Use rewards other than food

22. The adults in the family model good eating habits.
    a. yes   b. no
    *Goal: Children have strong role models to follow as they learn new eating
                             habits*

23. Our family caters to what children like to eat and does not require them to try new foods.
    a. true   b. false
    Goal: Encourage all who are present to try new food and eat what is served

24. My child talks negatively about his/her body.

   a. yes   b. no

   Goal: Self-talk should be positive and healthy

25. I think my child eats for emotional reasons.

   a. yes   b. no

   Goal: Eat when physically hungry, not for other unrelated reasons

Turning to New Habits

Great eating habits aren't hard to incorporate—if we follow the basics.

1. Eat to Satisfy Hunger and Nothing More

Physical hunger is different than eating out of boredom or other emotional needs. Physical hunger builds gradually and begins with a growling or rumbling stomach. Another indicator is the falling energy level most kids experience right before it's time to eat. Difficulty concentrating and increased irritability are also indicators of true physical hunger.

A significant problem with overweight kids is that many eat when they aren't hungry. Instead of satisfying hunger, eating fills up time or satisfies other needs. If your child eats for emotional reasons, you'll have to teach her new coping methods, which we will cover in chapter 8. Ask your child if she is really hungry or whether she feels bored, or if the food just sounds good.

If she doesn't know what real hunger is, teach her to pay attention to her body and describe what the symptoms of physical hunger are. In addition, pay attention to the time of her last meal or snack. If it has been three to four hours since her last meal, she is probably hungry. Young children get hungry after short intervals because their little tummies can only handle so much food at one time. If she isn't hungry, encourage her to wait until mealtime to eat, and then distract her with something else to do.

2. Stop Eating When Full

For those of us taught to clean our plates, this is a tough one. We still feel guilt over all those poor children in third-world countries who are starving because we waste food at the table! We need to let go of this whole method. Forcing kids to eat when they don't want to leads to big battles, and if waste is the issue, it's not a big deal to wrap up food and serve it for a snack at a later time. *If a person is full, the food is better left on the plate then eaten.* Kids know when they feel full unless they have a physical problem related to hunger.

> **TIP BOX #1**
>
> In order to help an overweight child avoid eating when she is not hungry, store food out of sight. If there are yummy brownies on the counter, she will be tempted to eat them—hunger or no hunger. If the brownies are wrapped in foil and stored in the freezer, they are less tempting. In fact, she probably won't even think about them. Out of sight, out of mind!

The same habits hold true when eating out. Since restaurant portions are usually large, tell your child the uneaten portion of the food will be wrapped up and taken home for a snack later when he is hungry again. He should feel free to stop eating when he is full.

3. Eat at the Table

Early in life, teach your children that eating happens at the table during mealtimes, not while watching television and unconsciously putting food in your mouth. Sure, it's fine to put up the TV trays and eat during a special movie once in a while, but not very often! Food should be eaten during mealtimes, at the table, whether in the kitchen or dining room. (Notice I didn't say you should eat in the car, in front of the morning news, or while reading, surfing the Internet, or while attending church!) All of this eating everywhere and anytime is not helping us establish good habits.

We are so pressed for time that it seems like mealtimes are when we catch up on light activities. This is a bad idea. When we spend our dining moments stressing over the bills we are opening, or checking the stock market figures, or watching the news, we don't pay any attention to what we are eating or how much we are eating, or even whether or not we are full.

4. Schedule Mealtimes

There is no substitute for consistency when it comes to instilling good eating habits in our children. Too often the family meal is given little or no priority as other pressing events dictate what the family's evening will look like. You know what I mean—soccer games, ballet practice, late business meetings, church functions, piano lessons, and whatever other activities are on the calendar.

The breakdown of regular family mealtimes is a sad result of the changing face of the family as we know it. We are too busy to sit down for twenty minutes with the people we are closest to, even when the goal is to enjoy some good food and good company. Yet when there is a regular dinnertime, there tend to be regular snack times and better expectations in place for when and what children are to eat. This step cannot be skipped if we want to improve our family's overall health when it comes to eating. Meals should be scheduled and everyone should participate. We'll discuss this more a little later in the book.

When you have meals, have your child come to the table. Even if your child insists he is not hungry, he must join the family. Don't force him to eat, but have him participate with the family in conversation and be present for the meal-time. Eating together is a special part of eating in general.

> **TIP BOX #3**
> Turn off the excess media during mealtimes, which includes the TV, computer, and even the radio! Make mealtimes more relaxing and give attention instead to the other people at the table.

5. Choose Healthy Food

Go through your pantry and get rid of all the junk food and unhealthy snacks. Then stock your pantry with better items such as baked low-fat chips, nuts, yogurt, and fruit. If the healthy foods are the only snacks, your kids will eat them. When I first did this with my kids, they would open the pantry door, stare at the options, and say, "Mom, there is nothing to eat." Then I would point out the food they didn't want to eat. For the first few weeks, they went without. Eventually, they started snacking on the healthier items, to the point that it was habitual and they didn't complain about the choices available.

> **TIP BOX #4**
> "Grazing" is a term dieticians use to describe continuous eating which occurs all day—picture cows grazing in a green field all day. I know this isn't a flattering description of how people eat, but it provides a great picture for the type of eating many people have fallen into. Grazing on food all day puts on weight, and though it's great for cows, it's not for people! It's a habit that can be kicked back to the hayfield with the use of regular, scheduled mealtimes.

Evaluate how you cook and try to make the food choices healthier. In place of baked products, make fruit and other low-calorie items dessert. At the end of the meal, put out an attractive-looking plate of berries, cut-up bananas, and other scrumptious fruit. If you want to make it a little more special, serve fruit with an angel food cake and low-fat Cool Whip and you've got a great dessert for kids. And though your family might tell you they *have* to have ice cream every night, or that they really want apple pie instead of baked apples, if you are persistent, new and healthier eating habits will form.

TIP BOX #5

Fresher, better, and more nutritious food begins at home. Cooking from scratch is not that hard, even with major time constraints. There are many wonderful recipe books available for tasty, healthy meals that don't use processed food or prepackaged items. Consider updating your cookbook selection to include a few new choices. Give the recipes I've included in appendix D a try, and buy a Crock-Pot to help simplify the entire process.

Cooking should not be left entirely up to the wife and mother, either! Men are equally capable when it comes to kitchen chores and food preparation; in truth, the whole family should be involved in meal preparation, from grocery shopping to cleanup.

Kids can be involved at every step. Grocery shopping is a great way to do on-site training. Since you are buying foods, you can discuss what you buy and why. Talk about your choices and how to avoid buying on impulse, but please don't shop when you are hungry. As to cooking, kids generally enjoy simple tasks like stirring the pasta, shredding lettuce for the salad, and grating cheese. Setting the table is another great task for kids. Encourage their participation. They will learn about nutrition and cooking while also spending time with you. And when it comes time to clean up the kitchen and clear the table, make it a family event so the task goes faster.

When your child eats healthy food, praise her. It's so important to praise behavior you want to encourage and ignore behavior you want to discourage. Positive attention for appropriate behavior is one of the best parenting strategies you can use when teaching your child new eating habits.

6. Allow Kids to Eat Treats

I've been to so many birthday parties at which mothers hover over their kids and say something like, "No, Sally doesn't want any birthday cake." Meanwhile, Sally looks longingly at the cake, heaves a big sigh, and sits by herself. By the look on Sally's face, I'll probably be seeing her in therapy someday. Don't do this. Let 'em eat cake!

Not that you should go crazy and stock your pantry with boxes of cake mixes (remember moderation?), but you shouldn't try and keep your child from enjoying a treat with the rest of the kids. When parents don't allow a child to indulge, the child puts a premium on that cake, thinks about it to the point of almost obsessing, and wants that cake enough that he will determine then and there to eat it when you aren't around. Eating cake at a party isn't going to put on the pounds . . . but eating cake at home for dessert every night just might.

The same goes for dining out. It's okay to indulge, but use

> **TIP BOX #6**
> It seems like I was constantly reminding my kids to slow down when it came to eating or running in the house. Kids often eat quickly because they are focused on an upcoming activity after the meal. This is a bad practice because eating quickly can cause people to overeat. Our stomachs haven't told our brains we are full yet. Consequently, we can stuff food down and then feel overly full after our brains have signaled us that we overate.

moderation when you do so. If you can avoid fast-food places, by all means, do. If your child is pleading and begging to go to McDonald's and it has been a month since you've indulged, why not go to McDonald's, but with the mindset of eating in moderation? No super-sizing, and what about sharing a box of fries between yourself and your child? And how about ordering milk instead of the soda?

7. Food Innovation

As kids grow older, their tastes can change. They may find out they like a certain food they passed up before. I remember the day we were all pleas-antly surprised when my daughter started eating salads. She wouldn't eat them before the age of nine. Now salads are a mainstay for her. Offer new and different foods regularly and encourage your child to take a bite and try them. It's best to introduce a new food with familiar favorites.

Even though food is delicious, it shouldn't be used as a punishment or reward. Eating vegetables is not a suitable punishment for being dis-respectful at the table. And eating an entire box of chocolates is not an acceptable reward for getting straight A's this semester. When foods are used as a punishment or reward, the child puts a higher value on them, which can actually increase the child's desire to eat more and more of those particular items.

The Quick Fix for Healthy Snacks

You don't have to be wildly creative or spend a lot of time on preparation to offer healthy, nutritious, and great-tasting snacks. Check out these possibilities if you need to infuse some new snack habits. Keep in mind that children prefer foods that are presented in fun and interesting ways. Any time you can use a fun cup, dish, straw, or spoon, or cut something up with a cookie cutter or interesting shape, do it! Use a melon baller to make circles, or skewer food on a toothpick (remove before they eat it)—whatever gets their attention. Also, toddlers and preschoolers (ages

1–6) only need small portions to have a healthy snack—the rule of thumb for children's serving sizes are usually one tablespoon for each year of age.

TIP BOX # 7

Eating breakfast is so important for our health. Even though some kids would prefer to skip this meal, parents should be firm. If gaining compliance means adding variety to the choices for this first and very important meal of the day, so be it.

Even though my daughter hates to eat breakfast, she is required to eat in the morning, because if she doesn't she'll overeat at lunch from being so hungry. And it isn't good for her to start her day on an empty stomach. Most kids become tired and cranky when they haven't eaten all night or in the morning. Kids don't think well on an empty stomach, either. As parents, we need to make sure our children are ready to study and learn, and that means eating breakfast.

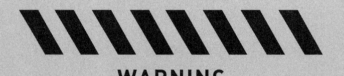

WARNING

Children ages three and younger can choke on foods that aren't cut up into small pieces. Avoid raw vegetables, grapes, popcorn, nuts, and dried fruits as these are items that can cause choking.

Healthy Snacks

- Cut-up apples or celery to dip in peanut butter (look for natural peanut butter that doesn't contain trans fat); also can add raisins

- Low-fat or nonfat yogurt with fruit or low-fat granola added

- Low-fat or whole-grain crackers with low-fat cheese or hummus

- Graham crackers spread with low-fat yogurt and then frozen

- Trail mixes with sunflower or pumpkin seeds and nuts; soy nuts mixed with raisins and dried fruit

- Fresh vegetables like carrots, broccoli, celery, and pea pods with low-fat Ranch dressing for dipping

- Whole-wheat tortillas with melted low-fat cheese, fat-free beans, a thin slice of lean ham or turkey, and cream cheese or salad dressing all rolled up and cut into triangles

- English muffins or whole-grain bagel halves with pizza sauce, low-fat melted cheese, and any vegetable

- Fat-free puddings

- Fresh fruits and cheeses skewered on kabobs using toothpicks. Another alternative is to dice fruit to make a fruit salad and pour freshly squeezed orange juice or lemon zest over the fruit to give it a little tang.

- String cheese—it's just fun to pull apart and eat

- Baked chips, pretzels, and air-popped popcorn

- Use a melon baller to scoop watermelon, cantaloupe, and honeydew. Just the shape is exciting!

- Frozen fruit bars, frozen bananas, and frozen seedless green grapes

- Mini low-fat muffins with added carrots, bananas, blueberries, bran, or other fruits and vegetables. Bake, freeze, and use as needed.

- Dry whole-grain cereals like Cheerios™ and Quaker Squares™

- Pumpkin seeds are a special treat. Every October we cut up pumpkins, scoop out the seeds, wash them, spray a tray with cooking spray, and season the seeds with salt. Then we roast the seeds under a broiler till they are toasted brown. Then we seal them in a plastic bag. If they get soggy, just put them under the broiler for a few minutes and they will return to their crunchy state.

- Oatmeal is a great snack. Cook it up when you have time, refrigerate it, and spoon out one serving at a time. Top with brown sugar.

- Eggs that are either hardboiled or sliced and deviled with light mayonnaise and mustard

- Sweet potatoes sprinkled with pumpkin spice. Take a small sweet potato and microwave it for about six minutes and then open it up and sprinkle pumpkin spice, cinnamon, or a small amount of brown sugar on it.

- Small baked potato with low-fat cheese and vegetables

- Shakes with low-fat milk, soy milk, or yogurt and fruit. Use a cup of skim milk, yogurt, or soy milk (you can even use soft tofu), ice cubes, fruit, and a dash of cinnamon, nutmeg, or vanilla. Place all ingredients in a blender and mix well.

- Homemade oatmeal cookies made with applesauce and less sugar; also Fig Newton bars and animal crackers

- Peanut butter and jelly sandwiches made with natural low-fat peanut butter, low-sugar jelly, and whole-grain bread

- Frozen orange cream Popsicles made with orange juice, water, and yogurt

- Pita bread with low-fat cheeses, lean meats, bean sprouts, and other vegetables

Making small changes yields big results over time. We can prevent our overweight kids from becoming overweight adults. If eating habits are gradually adjusted, the change will be less difficult to keep in place long-term. So approach this lifestyle change one eating habit at a time, and get ready to see the results!

POINTS TO PONDER

1. Avoid diets for kids—they don't work.

2. By becoming the food police, parents don't help a child become personally responsible for their health and well-being. Instead, parents should strive to teach children to make good food choices.

3. Balance and moderation are the keys to healthy eating and dining, and these are lessons learned best from parents, a child's most important role models.

4. Good eating habits begin at home. As a family, commit to healthier eating through better food choices and the act of sharing meals together. The effort is so worth the results!

4

The Do's and Don'ts of Eating Habits

Though we live in a land of abundance, eating well can become an exhausting goal. On our own, we can easily become worn out and worn down while trying to offer healthy, nutritious food. Have you heard any lines similar to these?

"Mom, it's only a soda. What's wrong with me having it right now? Please?"

"I saw this cereal on TV and it's awesome. Can we get it?"

"They eat doughnuts at Sarah's house for breakfast. Why can't we?"

"Please, please, please! Can I have the kid's meal? It's got the best toy."

After answering with ten no's in regard to eating candy for a snack, fighting traffic, running three errands, taking Jimmy to soccer, and arguing your claim with the insurance company over the phone, you find yourself relenting, "Alright. Whatever. Yes." After all, can eating candy for just one snack really do much harm? The answer is yes if a pattern emerges of giving in to what we know isn't helpful.

In terms of parenting, one of the best things parents can do for their children is tell them no. When kids want something that isn't in their best interest, parents need to be able to say no and stick with their answer. To a child, it will be frustrating, but also reassuring—*when Mom and Dad say no, they mean no.* Children who understand they can't manipulate their parents will grow to count on that strength instead of always trying to wear it down. Setting limits is like driving across a bridge with guard rails. Without the rails, the drive could be pretty scary. Limits put rails on the bridges of life, and when you use them, children feel more secure.

To succeed in advancing a healthier set of eating habits, you have to stick with your decision and not succumb to the requests for junk food, no matter what. Though the responsibility for raising healthy kids is shared by families, schools, and communities, your job as a parent is to provide *what* your kids eat and supervise *when* and *where* they eat it. The younger your child, the more control you have over which foods are offered. Two-year-olds can't run to a fast-food eatery and order fries . . . but you can. And four-year-olds aren't spending thirty-five hours a week at school and choosing to eat hot dogs and chips for lunch. Obviously, it's easier to supervise and monitor what a younger child eats than a teenager. Children between the ages of ten and fifteen have access to many foods outside the home, thus requiring them to make good choices somewhat independent of your direction. But our kids learn what to eat when they are young by watching our examples as parents. And even when they are teens, the breakfast and dinner we provide can be nutritious and influence what they choose for those meals when they aren't at home.

Parents aren't the only ones with responsibilities when it comes to healthy eating. Children must pay attention to how much they eat and whether or not they will eat certain foods. The training for this lesson begins at home . . . and once again, it's time to see how we parents are doing.

Take the Quiz

1. Do you talk to your kids about what they eat?
   YES   NO

2. Do you encourage them to eat with good health being the goal?
   YES   NO

3. Do you put out fruits and veggies for healthy snacking?
   YES   NO

4. Do you pack nutritious meals when they're on the go?
   YES   NO

5. Do you know what snacks they are eating after school?
   YES   NO

6. Do you set a good example in terms of what you eat?
   YES   NO

7. Is eating breakfast everyday important to your family?
   YES   NO

8. Is it a family priority to eat healthy dinners together?
   YES   NO

9. Is junk food readily available in your home?
   YES   NO

10. Are mealtimes scheduled, even if they vary from day to day?
    YES   NO

What to Eat

The following information regarding what children eat is put out by the Center for Science in the Public Interest:[1]

Ten of the Worst Foods for Children:

1. Soda pop
2. Whole milk (over two years of age)
3. Hamburgers
4. American cheese
5. Hot dogs
6. French fries and tater tots
7. Ice cream
8. Pizza loaded with cheese and meat
9. Bologna
10. Chocolate bars

Ten of the Best Foods for Children:

1. Fresh fruits and vegetables (especially carrot sticks, cantaloupe, watermelon, and strawberries)
2. Chicken breasts and drumsticks without skin or breading
3. Cheerios™, Wheaties™, or other whole-grain, low-sugar cereals
4. Skim or 1 percent milk
5. Extra lean ground beef or vegetarian burgers (Garden Burgers™ or Green Giant Harvest Burgers™
6. Low-fat hot dogs (Yves Veggie Cuisines Fat-free Wieners™ or Lightlife Fat-free Smart Dogs™
7. Nonfat ice cream or frozen yogurt
8. Fat-free corn chips or potato chips
9. Seasoned air-popped popcorn
10. Whole-wheat crackers or Small World Animal Crackers™

If you are ready to panic because your kids eat items off the first list, hang on! You can gradually make changes. Begin by replacing one food item at a time with a healthy substitute version of that food, or eliminate the food altogether. When you make changes gradually, your kids may not even notice. For example, when both of my children were over two years old, I made gradual changes with the milk. First I bought 2 percent, then 1 percent, and then skim. My kids really didn't like skim milk for drinking, but they didn't mind 1 percent. They do use skim milk on their cereal because there isn't as much of a taste difference.

In terms of what children eat, food choices either help or hinder healthy growth of their developing bodies. Unfortunately, a majority of parents are choosing less than ideal foods for their children. The Gerber Products Company commissioned a study involving more than 3,000 youngsters between the ages of four months and two years old. In the study, parents were randomly called and asked what they fed their child in the previous 24 hours. Based on the parents' reporting, the study indicated what specific foods were consumed. The research yielded the following discovery: children in this age range are being fed as well as overfed the wrong types of food. Here are a few of the specifics taken from the *USA Today* article summarizing the study. Again, the study was for children between four months and two years old.

- Up to one-third of the children ate no fruits or vegetables. Those who did reported french fries as the most common vegetable given to children 15 months of age and older.

- Fries were eaten at least once a day by 9 percent of children 9–11 months old. Twenty percent of children between 19 months and 2 years old ate fries every day.

- Hot dogs, sausage, and bacon also were eaten on a daily basis for many children: seven percent in the 9- to 11-months-old group, and 25 percent in the older range.

- Dessert and candy were eaten by more than 60 percent of kids 12 months old at least once per day; 16 percent ate a salty snack. Those numbers shot up to 70 percent and 27 percent by children 19 months of age.

- Sugary fruit drinks were downed daily by 30–40 percent of children ages 15 months and older.

- Soda was consumed by about 10 percent of the kids aged 15 months and older on a daily basis.

Interestingly, most of these foods are on the list of worst foods. The study involved young children who depend solely on their parents to provide healthy foods. A Chicago dietitian, Jodie Shield, had this to say about the study: "If kids are having soda and soft drinks at such an early age, it's going to be very, very challenging to introduce other types of foods for them later."[2]

When Is a Good Time?

Babies are born with a preference for sweets and develop a preference for salt at around four months of age, but all other tastes are learned. So once a child is eating solid food, it is wise to begin to introduce him to a variety of foods. There is evidence to suggest that the sooner babies are exposed to new foods, the more likely they are to accept new foods later in life.[3]

Introduce new foods one at a time. Wait to see if your child has an allergic reaction to a food before you introduce another. Keep in mind that kids learn to like foods that are made available to them. Keep the portion small. Sometimes, it can take 10–20 times of introducing a new food before your toddler will try it. Be persistent, but don't criticize him if he resists. It isn't wise to push certain foods on your child either. Children are developing their personal tastes and likes and dislikes.

The Common Sense Approach to Eating

When you think about the changes that have taken place in food preparation over the past few years, it's no wonder that the *way* we eat and *what* we eat are causing problems. The most noted change is the move away from preparing food from scratch and instead using more pre-packaged, frozen meals and other processed food-stuffs. These convenient meal options are often filled with too many preservatives, unhealthy fats, sugars, and salt.

THE WAY WE EAT AND WHAT WE EAT ARE CAUSING PROBLEMS.

Kids today can make their own meals in the microwave and eat prepared food right out of the box. And while all of us moms are thankful for the added convenience that has made our lives easier, we need to rethink how much such changes affect the weight of our kids. Dieticians tell us we are eating more foods from the top of the food pyramid rather than those from the base.

There is a separate food pyramid on the following page for very young children between two and six years of age.[4]

Overall, the amount of calories a child needs depends on how well he burns energy, a factor which is influenced by a child's activity level, body size, age, and gender. The Mayo Clinic recommends that, on average, children need about 1,600 calories a day. Older children need around 2,200 calories, and teenage boys need approximately 2,800 calories.[5]

Though it might be tempting to start counting calories with our children, this activity isn't recommended. It tends to lead people to diet and can turn our kids into low-carb kids. We don't want to eliminate food groups in the name of cutting calories. Instead, we need to try to follow the recommended guidelines when it comes to feeding our children. Use your common sense. A healthy lifestyle is better than a short-lived diet or other unhealthy diet. Don't forget that little changes add up to big results over time. Here are some great suggestions to consider.

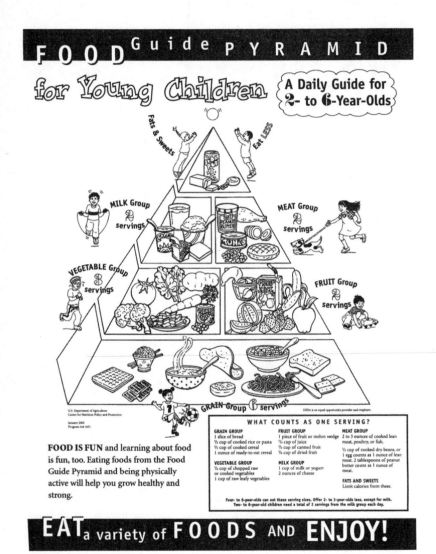

FOOD Guide PYRAMID

for Young Children

A Daily Guide for 2- to 6-Year-Olds

Fats & Sweets — Eat LESS

MILK Group
2 servings

MEAT Group
2 servings

VEGETABLE Group
3 servings

FRUIT Group
2 servings

GRAIN Group 6 servings

U.S. Department of Agriculture
Center for Nutrition Policy and Promotion

January 2000
Program Aid 1651

USDA is an equal opportunity provider and employer.

FOOD IS FUN and learning about food is fun, too. Eating foods from the Food Guide Pyramid and being physically active will help you grow healthy and strong.

WHAT COUNTS AS ONE SERVING?

GRAIN GROUP
1 slice of bread
½ cup of cooked rice or pasta
½ cup of cooked cereal
1 ounce of ready-to-eat cereal

VEGETABLE GROUP
½ cup of chopped raw or cooked vegetables
1 cup of raw leafy vegetables

FRUIT GROUP
1 piece of fruit or melon wedge
¾ cup of juice
½ cup of canned fruit
¼ cup of dried fruit

MILK GROUP
1 cup of milk or yogurt
2 ounces of cheese

MEAT GROUP
2 to 3 ounces of cooked lean meat, poultry, or fish.

½ cup of cooked dry beans, or 1 egg counts as 1 ounce of lean meat. 2 tablespoons of peanut butter count as 1 ounce of meat.

FATS AND SWEETS
Limit calories from these.

Four- to 6-year-olds can eat these serving sizes. Offer 2- to 3-year-olds less, except for milk.
Two- to 6-year-old children need a total of 2 servings from the milk group each day.

EAT a variety of FOODS AND ENJOY!

Buy and eat more fresh fruits and vegetables. I know this can be a shopping pain because you have to go to the store more often in order to get and use fresh produce, but the extra effort is well worth your family's health. Fruits and vegetables make up the second layer of the food pyramid, yet these are the least eaten of all the food groups for many kids.

If your kids aren't wild about the fruit you serve, consider trying some new fruits. Let your children pick out the fruits and vegetables they like and want to try when you are grocery shopping. Who knew? My son likes mangos and enjoys picking them out at the store. In his mind, they are a bit exotic and more enticing to eat than apples and bananas. And since I know they are a healthy food choice, we're all happy.

It's also a good idea to have a fruit bowl sitting on the counter. Seeing the fruit stacked in an attractive bowl on the kitchen counter may encourage your child to eat it for snacks. For vegetables, pull out the low-fat Ranch dressing to use as a dip for snacking on fresh carrots or other vegetables.

Avoid soft drinks and other sugary drinks. Snacking on soda or sugary juice is a hefty addition to the recommended daily caloric intake. The average soda has 160 calories and 40 grams of sugar—and zero nutrition. These beverages actually do harm because of the sugar and caffeine involved. If you don't have soda in the house, kids will drink more milk and water instead.

Go low-fat. Low-fat is good when it comes to choosing dairy products. For example, use low-fat dressings on salads, and buy low-fat cheeses and milk for children older than age two. Do keep in mind that low-fat doesn't necessarily mean low-calorie. A product can be low-fat yet still have lots of sugar in it. Read labels.

As it pertains to cooking, keep looking for ways to cut out the fat. The average American eats the equivalent of one whole stick of butter a day.[6] If you grew up in a tradition in which everything was fried or covered with rich sauces, make changes in the way you cook. Poach, boil, and broil more often. Cooking sprays can also cut down on the fat.

Eliminate as much trans fat in your child's diet as you can. Trans fat occurs naturally in some foods, but most trans fat is added to improve texture and longevity of foods. This fat is produced by the partial hydrogenation of oils. You will see it listed on products as "partially hydrogenated," "shortening," "partially hydrogenated vegetable oil," or "hydrogenated vegetable oil." When you see this ingredient on a label, note if it comes near the top of the list of ingredients, because the higher it appears on the list, the more trans fat there is in the product. Trans fat is also specifically listed on the "Nutrition Facts" labels of foods. If you want to really help your family's health out, avoid buying products with this food ingredient. These "bad fats" contribute to heart disease and childhood diabetes.

Dr. Walter Willett is the chairman of the Department of Nutrition at the Harvard School of Public Health and professor of medicine at the Harvard Medical School. He considers trans fats to be ". . . the biggest food-processing disaster in U.S. history."[7] And about 40 percent of food that is on the grocery store shelves—like cookies, crackers, and microwave popcorn—contain trans fat![8] Once I realized that microwave popcorn contained trans fat, I went back to popping popcorn the old-fashioned way. It takes a little more time and is less convenient, but the fact that I'm avoiding trans fat makes it worth it.

Increase fiber in your child's diet. The American Heart Association suggests that for children ages two and above, a "5 + age" guideline for fiber intake be used. To follow this guideline means you take the age of your child in addition to five extra grams of fiber in order to find how much fiber is right for your child. For an eight-year-old child, you would want that child to get thirteen grams of fiber a day (8+5=13).[9] Fiber helps a child with regularity and contributes to good health. A good source for fiber is fruits and vegetables and whole-grain cereals—which are all found on the two bottom tiers of the food pyramid!

Use less salt. You may want to remove the salt shaker from the table, because the more salt kids pile on their food, the more they want to add it. Preschoolers should have a low salt intake, and school age kids should

Good-bye, Fast Food

That's right, no more fast food. Unless you go for something like a healthy sub sandwich, fast-food restaurants are to be avoided. If you can't seem to cut out all fast food, try to cut back to only one meal a week. Making this change alone will really help your child. Along the same line, say no to supersizing. The original McDonald's meal (burger, fries, and twelve-ounce Coke) tallied up to 590 calories. Today's supersized extra value meal with a quarter-pound burger with cheese, fries, and soda has a whopping 1,550 calories![10]

If you have to eat fast food, order a regular or junior-size of an item in order to keep the portion size reasonable. Another option is to order individual burgers for everyone and then share a single container of fries. And if healthy options are given, such as substituting a salad or soup for fries, make the most of them!

When you ask for smaller portions, be prepared to defend your decision to persuasive servers. I once asked for a small drink at a fast-food restaurant and practically got into a fight with the person at the window. The young server kept insisting I wasn't getting the best deal. I got the concept that for twenty-five cents more I could have a bigger drink, but I didn't want a bigger drink—and this person didn't seem to care. It was a lesson in assertiveness training! Learn to say no and stick with your original request.

not have more than four grams per day. If you look at the salt levels of fast food, you will see that popular items like pizza and burgers have about half the daily recommendation![11]

Don't forget the calcium. This is important for the development of strong bones. Calcium can be found in milk, fortified juices, broccoli, mustard greens, kale, collard greens, northern beans, navy and baked beans, low-fat cheeses, yogurt, and no-fat ice cream. The recommendation is that preschoolers get between 500-800 milligrams (mg) of calcium a day; school age children need around 800 mg; and adolescents should have around 1,200–1,500 mg.[12] If you think your child isn't getting enough calcium each day, you may want to supplement with a popular calcium chew. If your child has a milk allergy, check to see if the calcium chew has milk in it.

Cut down on sugar. The average person in North America consumes twenty to thirty teaspoons of sugar a day, which means we have some work to do![13] While much of our sugar intake comes from soft drinks, sugar is the leading additive in foods. It's in all kinds of foods you wouldn't suspect, such as soups, yogurts, canned vegetables, and more. Candy, of course, is full of sugar. If it's available, kids will eat it. On holidays, it's especially plentiful, but parents can choose not to keep it in their own homes, which will help limit how much candy your child will be able to eat.

Drink more water. Most of us don't get enough water each day. Children need six to eight glasses of water a day, just like adults. When I say "glasses" I mean the eight-ounce size—for a total of between forty-eight and sixty-four ounces of water per day. Don't hesitate to serve water with meals or as a thirst quencher during the day. The more water they drink, the less soda they'll take in, and the healthier they'll be. Drink water at meals, and if you want some zing, add a wedge of lemon. And water is still the best quenching drink, so pack it instead of a sugary alternative.

> **TIP BOX #8**
>
> The extra calories that come with types of food that are doubled-up should be avoided. Cheesy fries will be more fattening than regular fries. The same is true about the deep-fried twinkie, stuffed crust pizza, and peanut butter-filled pretzels. If you need a treat, don't go with one of the doubled-up variety.

Foods to Increase	Foods to Decrease or Eliminate
fruits and vegetables	sugared and soft drinks
low-fat dairy products	fast food
fiber (use the 5 + age rule)	fat and trans fat
calcium	salt and sugar
water	stuffed or loaded "double" items

By making these dietary changes, the extra calories that contribute to weight gain above and beyond what is normally expected for a child will be minimized. And developing healthier eating habits will eliminate extra calories without having to count them. Making small changes adds up to big weight loss in a year's time![14]

Extra Weight Gained Last Year (in pounds)	Number of Calories to Eliminate Each Day
1	10
5	50
10	100
15	150
20	200
25	250
30	300

When to Eat

Food can be had and seen just about everywhere. Kids are used to seeing it at drug counters, gas stations, schools, and even the doctor's office. I've even visited churches that have food courts in them! Kids are conditioned to see food and want it.

The other day I took my daughter to the doctor. While we were waiting for the appointment, she opened a small bag which had a toy in it. A three-year-old boy walked by, pointed at the bag, and yelled, "I want cookies! See cookies, want cookies!" Just the sight of the bag evoked a response from this young child . . . and it didn't even have any cookies in it. The whole scene was more than a little surprising. The poor mom couldn't make him stop and ended up dragging him out of our sight. I wanted to open the bag and yell, "Look, no food!"

We have to break these conditioned responses that call for our children to have food whenever they want it. One way to do that is to teach children that eating happens at dining tables during specific times of the day. Generally speaking, there should be three meals a day with two snacks in between. Eating should occur in an orderly fashion. Try to avoid eating in the car and on the run. Another place to stop eating food would be in movie theaters and at home in front of the television. Eating should not be a form of "fun" or relaxation of and in itself. Establishing regular times helps to eliminate grazing and all-day snacking.

The Family Meal

I know times have changed and we can't go back to the 1950s (some of you are saying, "thank goodness!") but we can reinstate one holdover from days gone by—the family meal. Though *The Brady Bunch* and other similar shows from bygone eras may seem a little sappy in the new millennium, one thing they did right was to eat meals together as a family. Kids need this habit-forming activity from an early age if they want to learn to eat at the proper time—when everyone else is eating, during mealtimes. It's time to revive family dinners and put an end to what feels like a revolving family restaurant in which people come and go all times of the day and eat whatever they want.

Even when both parents work and kids play sports, it is possible to have a family meal if you make it a priority. Most of my families from clinical practice who had a child with an eating disorder did not eat meals together. Certainly food for thought, isn't it?

Research tells us that implementing regular family meals is tied to a decrease in teen risk of psychosocial problems, drug use, risky sexual behavior, and suicidal intention. Hey, that's enough incentive for me! And, not surprisingly, children who eat with their parents tend to eat healthier diets.[15]

EVEN WHEN BOTH PARENTS WORK AND KIDS PLAY SPORTS, IT IS POSSIBLE TO HAVE A FAMILY MEAL.

The dinner table is NOT the place for arguments, stressful discussions, or criticism of your child's grades, life, or clothing choices. Make mealtimes a stress-free zone. If you need further evidence to drive this point home, here it is: people who suffer eating disorders associate eating with stressful family meals and people. When and if they did eat family meals, mealtimes were tense and stressful because of the lack of emotional connection and unresolved family stress.

Revive the family meal and make it a priority for all involved. Look at your family's schedule and adjust the mealtime accordingly for each day, sometimes eating earlier or later in order to accommodate the various activities scheduled. You may even want to rethink the family schedule if you feel you are overscheduled. If you don't have even one day to eat at least one meal together, your family is too busy!

Meals should be associated with a relaxed, pleasant time. Good food is a pleasure, and so is good company. Work at making conversation lively and interesting. Ask about your child's day. Tell a funny story. Engage on an emotional level with your child so he won't have to engage on an emotional level with the food being served. Mealtimes are a great time to interact with one another and to enjoy a few minutes of peace and relaxation.

MEALTIMES ARE A GREAT TIME TO INTERACT WITH ONE ANOTHER AND TO ENJOY A FEW MINUTES OF PEACE AND RELAXATION.

Along the same line, build a routine into your mealtimes. The more routine meals are, the easier it will be to keep up family involvement. Another reason: kids thrive on schedules and predictability. If kids know what is expected in terms of how they are to help with preparation for the meal or cleanup, the whole event goes better.

Once you've decided the meal schedule for each day, stick to it. Then plan ahead for the actual meal. Try to decrease the number of processed foods and prepackaged meals you use and instead cook healthier foods. Use a Crock-Pot so food can slow-cook all day and be served when you get home. Utilize easy-to-prepare recipes that only take twenty minutes to fix. Cook ahead on the weekends and freeze meals that can be thawed on a daily basis. If you can afford it on really busy days, stop by a take-out that prepares healthy and fresh meals when you are short on time, or have them delivered to your home. Preplanning a daily menu and preparing food ahead takes pressure off you and helps the family stick to the goal of healthier eating.

One study shows that children who have regular dinners with their families had healthier dietary patterns in terms of the food they ate. Children who were studied (ages 9–14) ate more fruits and vegetables, less saturated fats, fewer fried foods, and even drank fewer sodas.[16]

If you still aren't convinced of the importance of the family meal, consider the results of this study conducted by the University of

Michigan. The single strongest predictor of better achievement scores and fewer behavioral problems was found with children who spent more mealtimes at home with their parents.[17]

Another important reason to revive family meals is because it sets a precedent and will evolve into a regular routine in the future. Research indicates that there is a strong association for teens between regular family meals (five or more dinners per week with a parent) and academic success, psychological adjustment, and lower rates of alcohol use, drug use, early sexual behavior, and suicidal risk. These results held for both single- and two-parent families.[18] The benefits are just too many to pass up when it comes to reinstating the family mealtime.

Eating Out

Even if it isn't a fast-food restaurant, parents need to know how to keep an overweight child on track when eating out. The portions at restaurants and fast-food joints are too large. The soft drinks flow too freely and the bread and appetizers are almost a meal in and of themselves. A few dining savvy tips to implement:

- Ask the waiter to bring you water right away. Encourage your child to drink water while waiting for the food to arrive. Say no to soft drinks and sugary juices.

- Tell the waiter to forgo the bread bowl, chips, or other calorie-laden yummies served before the meal.

- Encourage your child to order a salad or other vegetable with the meal instead of french fries.

- If the kids' meals are full of fried, fatty, and poor nutritional food, order an appetizer for your child's meal or split a meal from the adult menu. Avoid creamy sauces and buttery dishes.

- Rather than eating the entire meal, encourage your child to stop when he or she is full and have the rest of the meal wrapped up to take home.

- Suggest your child try a sandwich with mustard, vegetables, or salsa instead of mayonnaise.

- Go to salad bars and steer kids toward low-fat dressings and fresh fruits and vegetables instead of the high-fat cheeses, croutons, bacon bits, and mayonnaise-based dressings.

- Order fresh fruits for desserts.

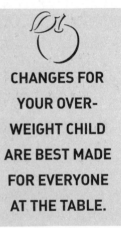

CHANGES FOR YOUR OVER-WEIGHT CHILD ARE BEST MADE FOR EVERYONE AT THE TABLE.

We covered a lot of ground in this chapter. If you follow these guidelines and make good choices in terms of what your child eats, you will go a long way to helping your overweight child. It takes time to change the way we eat, cook healthier meals, and structure our lives, but the end result is so worth it. Even after only a month, it gets easier and more natural to make changes in our eating habits. But it takes a commitment to prioritize the health and welfare of our families. Ready to give it a try?

POINTS TO PONDER

1. Parents provide the what, when, and where of eating.

2. The food pyramid for young children is an excellent resource in order to evaluate how many servings of the various food groups are recommended.

3. A common sense approach to eating will address problem areas in our eating habits and also encourage a lasting plan for a healthy lifestyle.

4. The benefits of eating meals together as a family far outweigh the scheduling difficulties . . . this is perhaps the easiest, most pain-free change to make.

5

Eat to Grow . . . Grow to Eat?

I'm so frustrated. My child cries for juice all the time. He just stands there and says, "Juice, juice." I'm not sure if I should give him juice every time he asks. I do use 100% juice, but as he is just two years old, drinking cups and cups of juice every day may not be a good thing. Is it?

I've heard you can overfeed an infant. Is that true? Some people say to put your infant on a feeding schedule; others say to feed her when she's hungry. What's right?

My three-year-old son doesn't want to come to the table to eat. My husband thinks he should sit quietly for the entire family meal. He squirms and is up and down at the table, making our mealtimes tense. Should we insist he stay at the table?

My preschooler is a picky eater. I've tried giving her a variety of foods, but she won't eat anything but macaroni and cheese. This can't be good for her. What should I do?

My ten-year-old son loves to eat and watch TV. Because our lives are so busy, he eats in front of the TV often. It doesn't seem like a big deal, but I notice he's gaining more weight.

We parents want our children to be healthy and to fit in with their peers. And while I hate to use the word *normal* to describe children since it implies abnormality when our children don't precisely do what other children their age are doing, it is helpful to know what other children we consider healthy are doing, what the typical pattern of weight gain and growth is for children, and what their eating habits are. Yet we must have a concept for what is expected behavior and what is not.

It helps us to have guidelines. Feeding issues can be unique to a child's developmental stage, and parents should know that what holds for a seven-year-old often doesn't hold for a three-year-old. Children go through so many stages of growth and eating habits that it's impossible to deal with all ages in exactly the same fashion. And so we will cover basic information about growth, development, and feeding according to specific age ranges for our children. The information here provides a general guide so that parents have a broad overview to know the variations in growth patterns that are common in kids as they grow from babies to teens.

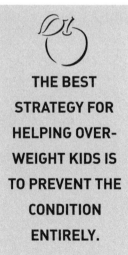

THE BEST STRATEGY FOR HELPING OVER-WEIGHT KIDS IS TO PREVENT THE CONDITION ENTIRELY.

Before Conception

Before I had a baby, I did everything in my power to prepare my body for conception. The reason I was so motivated was because I struggled with infertility for seven years. In the process of trying to become pregnant, I ate right, exercised, and kept myself physically fit. I couldn't control the infertility, but I could prepare my body for potential birth. As it turns out, my efforts were good for the baby!

The best strategy for helping overweight kids is to prevent the condition entirely. In fact, you can help a child with his weight before he's even born. Yes, you read that right. Prevention begins before conception! A mother-to-be should try to reach her ideal weight range before she decides to have a baby. I know this sounds a bit idealistic, but trying to be at a healthy weight before pregnancy *does* make a difference. And notice I used the word *trying.*

Consider this new finding from a study within an Ohio welfare program that looked at children and their moms: children born to obese moms were more than twice as likely to be overweight by age four.[1] Whether this study's findings can be applied to all moms is yet to be decided, but we do know that children with obese parents have an increased risk of becoming overweight. *So if you maintain a healthy weight, it helps your baby before she is even conceived.*

So you're thinking, *Great. That information will help me with future kids, but what about the ones I already have? I wasn't at a good weight when my daughter was conceived.* Don't worry about it. Changes can be made that will help you raise a healthy-weight child right now. So there is no condemnation if you are starting a little later. What is important is to recognize that you, Mom and Dad, are such an important part of your child's life!

In addition to being a healthy weight, moms need to have pregnancies free from exposure to alcohol, tobacco, drugs, and HIV. If you are thinking about becoming pregnant and have problems in any of these areas, please get help before you conceive so you can give your baby the best start possible. The more you take care of your own body before you conceive, the more it will help your baby in the long run.

The First Year

When we think about babies, we picture chubby little legs and cheeks that just beg to be squeezed and held tight. We smile when we see a round, fat baby. But a fat baby isn't necessarily a healthy baby, especially when obesity runs in a family. And we can't always assume that children will lose their baby fat as they get older. Many do, although there is disagreement on when that should happen. Some experts say around age six, and others say by age eight.[2]

During the first year of life, most infants gain about fifteen pounds in addition to what they weighed at birth. If you are thinking about "Cousin Jake" who weighed thirty pounds at age one and didn't turn out to be overweight, hold on to that thought. Gaining more than fifteen pounds doesn't mean you are doomed to be overweight later, but it does increase your risk. Remember, I'm speaking generally.

However, you may want to rethink the family story about Cousin Jake. There were the relatives who were concerned that Jake's mom fed him a bottle every time he cried when he was a baby. Remember how he struggled with his weight, losing and gaining the same twenty pounds all of his adult life? He complained that he had to be vigilant about his weight or he would gain too easily. So Jake did have weight struggles most of his life . . . and according to the growth charts, he was an overweight baby, falling above the 95th percentile.

It is possible to overfeed a baby, and it is medically proven that an infant who gains weight too quickly could have weight problems later in life. A study conducted by the Children's Hospital of Philadelphia and the University of Pennsylvania School of Medicine found that regardless of birth weight and weight at one year of age, infants who rapidly gained weight during the first four months of life had an increased risk of being overweight at age seven.[3] The reason may be because this is when the biological mechanisms that regulate obesity develop. The thinking of some researchers is that if you overfeed an infant baby formula or introduce solid carbohydrates too soon, you contribute to weight gain later in life.

Infants cry when they are hungry for milk, but they also cry when they are thirsty for water or want to be comforted or cuddled. If you always stick a bottle in a baby's mouth to comfort her, she may learn to associate food with comfort. Therefore, it is important to discern a baby's specific need before feeding. And often a baby who wants to suck can be appeased with a pacifier or his thumb.

What parents feed their infant can impact the baby later in life. The American Academy of Pediatrics recommends breastfeeding infants for the first year of life. There is good reason for this when it comes to a baby's weight—medical studies tell us that breastfeeding may prevent teen and adult obesity.[4] Breastfed babies tend to be leaner in the long run than formula-fed infants. This is believed in part to be a result of the frequency of breastfeeding. Infants allowed to nurse on cue (when they need to), rather than being put on a schedule, take in only the calories they need. This may be one reason they are leaner later in life—early on they learn to self-regulate their food intake and stop eating when they are full.[5]

Infants who are fed formula with bottles should not be encouraged to finish the entire bottle just for the sake of emptying the bottle. Babies know what they need in the way of food and will stop eating when they are full. It is also not necessary to widen the hole in the nipple so the baby can take in more formula faster. The baby should take her time with the designed nipple. Like an adult, there is a need to slow down while eating in order to experience the sensation of fullness which tells us to stop eating. If infants feed too quickly, they can't regulate their intake effectively. And if your baby sleeps through a scheduled feeding time, it isn't necessary to wake her up because it is time to feed. She can eat when she wakes up, and no harm will be done.

All babies are born with a preference for sweets. That's right, the desire for sweets (chocolate, in my case!) are built into our bodies from the very beginning. Yet even though this preference for sweets is innate, it doesn't mean we should feed infants chocolate

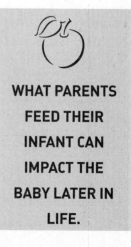

WHAT PARENTS FEED THEIR INFANT CAN IMPACT THE BABY LATER IN LIFE.

or other sweet treats, such as juice. Though juice is made from fruit, in reality this substance is a source of empty calories, like liquid candy, and it's bad for a baby's teeth. Water is a much better choice if you want to give your infant something besides breast milk or formula.

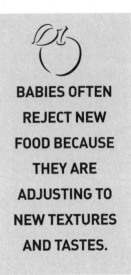

By the time babies reach four months old, they also develop a preference for salt. Other than salty and sweet, all other tastes are learned. When babies begin to eat solid foods, exposure to new foods is very important because their tastes are forming. New foods should be introduced one at a time, beginning with rice cereal. A serving for a small baby is between one and three tablespoons' worth. You should wait to see if your baby has an allergic reaction to one food before you introduce another.

BABIES OFTEN REJECT NEW FOOD BECAUSE THEY ARE ADJUSTING TO NEW TEXTURES AND TASTES.

If you've ever seen a baby try a new food, you know what happens when she's less than pleased. She'll turn away, spit out the food and act

FEEDING THE BABY[6]

What Baby Should Eat	When It's Time
Rice cereal mixed with breast milk or formula	Around 6 months old, or when baby is ready
Barley or oat cereal, followed by wheat or mixed grain cereal	2–3 weeks after introducing rice cereal
Vegetables: green beans, peas, carrots, squash, etc.	2–3 weeks after other cereals were introduced
Fruits: pears, apples, peaches, bananas, berries, etc.	2–3 weeks after veggies were introduced
Meats: chicken, beef, pork	2–3 weeks after fruits were introduced

Ready Yet?

It's important not to feed a baby solid food too quickly as this may cause food allergies and eczema later. General advice is that most babies aren't ready for solid foods until six months of age. One marker of a child's readiness for solid food is her ability to sit up. Another is her ability to hold her head up easily. The first solid food to introduce is rice cereal mixed with breast milk or formula.

like you've just fed her something awful. Babies often will reject new food because they are adjusting to new textures and tastes. Therefore, it is necessary to expose babies to new foods over and over. So don't give up; one day she may actually eat those red beets rather than spit them all over the table!

Between One and Two Years Old

Between the ages of twelve and twenty-four months, most breastfed babies are off the breast and transitioning to a routine which includes three meals a day. Regular meals and snacks should be scheduled and a wide variety of foods offered. Babies at twelve months of age will allow you to feed them even as they are eager to be active and moving—proof of continuously developing motor skills.

Around fifteen months, babies often want to feed themselves. Life gets messier at this point, but try to see your child's newfound independence as a good thing. By eighteen months or so, a baby's appetite may decrease, although most babies will eat food offered to them. Around twenty-one months, toddlers begin to show more food preferences. This is a great age to get in the habit of avoiding overly sugary, salty, or high-fat foods.

As long as your toddler is active and within the normal range for weight, the quantity of food he consumes is less of an issue than the

Personality Matters

According to well-known pediatrician Dr. William Sears, author of *The Baby Book,* diet isn't the only thing that influences weight gain. A child's temperament can also influence his eating. Dr. Sears says that a more driven, active infant burns more calories than a laid back, mellow type. Also, longer, leaner babies metabolize food faster than plump babies.[7]

quality. Children this age lose interest in food when distracted by activity and also when they don't feel well. Kids get colds, throat infections, and other ailments that decrease their appetite, but usually toddlers will respond to their body's need for energy and eat when they are truly hungry.

If your child is overweight, consider the portion size and what specific foods she is consuming. Usually the culprit is too much fat, sugar, or salt and not enough fruits and vegetables. Dieting is not the answer. Young children this age need all the nutrients they get from food to help their bodies grow healthy. Toddlers are just beginning to cultivate personal tastes, and they learn to like foods that are made available to them. When offering a new food to a toddler, keep the portion small and offer a single-ingredient food at a time. It can take ten to twenty repetitions of introducing a new food before your toddler will try it. So persist! If she resists, don't criticize or push certain foods on your child. Instead, make mealtime fun. Experiment with sauces and dips, keeping in mind that these tiny tots are developing their eating habits and need to be encouraged to eat healthy. They will probably give certain foods a dirty look. Such behavior is to be expected as they are simply developing their tastes. Children learn to associate foods with experiences that are positive or negative. If you threaten them with vegetables and reward them with sweets, vegetables become the enemy and sweets become the cherished prize. Food should not be used as a reward. Instead, food should be associated with keeping their body healthy and giving it the energy it needs to function well.

Food should not be treated as a distraction. Sitting kids in front of a TV with a plate loaded with snacks so you can get something done establishes an early habit of watching TV and eating. You don't want to encourage this. A better strategy is to give your child something to play with that will keep him distracted. When you finish your task, sit down with your child and have a scheduled snack.

Mealtimes should be relaxed and not a time of power struggles. Toddlers will eat if they are hungry. It's not recommended to insist they clean their plate or finish a jar of baby food—if they are full they will stop eating, in which case they shouldn't have to eat more. Foods at this stage should be soft, cut into small pieces, and relatively easy to chew.

When you present a healthy food that your toddler doesn't like, try serving it again when she is really hungry. According to dietitian and pediatrician Barbara Kolp-Jurss, most children taste a food eight times before they accept it.[8] So don't get discouraged if your child scrunches up her nose at the mashed peas on her plate. Continue to offer mashed peas and suggest she try a bite.

As far as beverages go, when children learn to hold a cup, which generally happens around a year of age (though sometimes earlier), offer milk at snacks and mealtimes. It's fine to offer an early morning or late night bottle during the transition to the cup. Toddlers need about two to three cups of milk or milk substitutes a day, which may include yogurt and cheese. During their first two years of life, a baby's brain is growing rapidly and needs the fat in whole milk. Therefore, don't give a toddler skim or 1 or 2 percent milk before they reach the age of two.

For kids who really like to drink milk, it doesn't hurt to limit their intake to three cups a day so they don't fill up on milk and lose their appetite for other foods. They need all the nutrients in other foods as well, so offer water if they want more to drink. In terms of fruit juices, water is a better alternative. If you use fruit juice, use 100% fruit juice, in small amounts, and dilute it with water. Limit it to no more than six ounces a day. Too much juice can cause diarrhea, stomachaches, and tooth decay. And resist giving toddlers soda and other sugary drinks.

At this age, dieticians usually recommend four servings of fruits or vegetables a day.[9] The rule of thumb they use is this: a serving size is one tablespoon for every year of age. When you think about it, that really is a small amount of food. Four servings of bread and an iron-fortified cereal should be given, along with two servings of meat, eggs, peanut butter, or beans. Try to get your toddler to eat these portions throughout the week. It may not be easy at first, but work toward the goal of a balanced diet. Be careful not to be overly strict with food rules or indulge in junk foods as both activities increase cravings for food.

If your toddler begins to eat only a certain group of foods, keep offering all the groups from the food pyramid (see chapter 4). Each day, try four to eight tablespoons of fruits and vegetables, four servings of breads and cereals, and two servings of meat, poultry, eggs, or legumes. Keep mixing things up so she experiences variety in her food choices, but keep in mind that her appetite at this age won't be huge because her growth rate is decreasing.

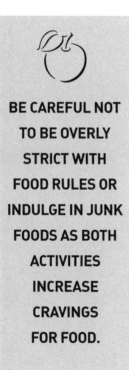

BE CAREFUL NOT TO BE OVERLY STRICT WITH FOOD RULES OR INDULGE IN JUNK FOODS AS BOTH ACTIVITIES INCREASE CRAVINGS FOR FOOD.

If you are a fanatic about being clean, you may need therapy at this stage of development! Things can get really messy when your child tries to feed herself. Thank goodness we had a dog to keep our floors clean. The best suggestion I can make is this: throw a drop cloth or vinyl tablecloth on the floor and let your child do her thing. Your child is showing initiative and working on her independence. Let it fly along with the food! Keep your child in the high chair as this is best for all concerned. And put the food right on the tray or you will spend lots of time picking up bowls and utensils.

Two- to Three-Year-Olds

Growth slows down a bit and so this age child doesn't need a very large amount of calories. Three-year-olds usually weigh between twenty-five and forty-four pounds and are thirty-four to forty-three inches tall.[10] They tend to have good appetites although you still may only get one good meal out of them. They are busy and social at this age. Their preferences are less pronounced and they enjoy eating meat, fruit, sweets, and milk. Vegetables can still be a challenge, but persevere and continue to present those greens at meals and snacks.

Kids this age sometimes become picky eaters or get locked into eating only certain foods. Don't worry, as this may be part of a growing independence. Few children this age get all their food requirements at each meal. If you are concerned that they aren't getting all the nutrition they need, add a daily vitamin to the mix.

Take another look at the food pyramid (see page 68). The base of the pyramid represents the bread, cereal, rice, and pasta group—the food group kids ages 2–6 years are supposed to eat roughly six servings from each day. Fruits and vegetables are next up with three servings of vegetables and two of fruit being recommended each day.

Next come the meat and dairy groups. Kids need two servings from the meat, poultry, eggs, fish, dry beans, and nuts group. From the dairy group, kids should try to eat two servings total of milk, yogurt, or cheese. At the very top of the pyramid are the fats, oils, and sweets—with the recommendation that these foods be used sparingly.

This is an active age when feeding patterns are usually established in a child for life. One of your most important goals is to teach your child to stop eating when she is full, which means not insisting that children clean their plates. It's more important for kids to stop eating when they are full. Understandably, children are more interested in play at this stage, which means they have limited attention spans for sitting still at the table. My advice is to not make the table a battleground. A child this age can spot an uptight grown-up in a minute and make mealtime unpleasant. Don't let that happen. Go with the flow. Let them eat and leave; they can learn to properly sit through the entire mealtime a little later in their development.

Make food preparation a fun experience. Two-year-olds can tear foods like lettuce and salad ingredients, and three-year-olds can stir many ingredients together. Have them help you shop and prepare meals.

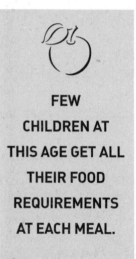

FEW CHILDREN AT THIS AGE GET ALL THEIR FOOD REQUIREMENTS AT EACH MEAL.

During this age period, a child's diet actually begins to resemble the rest of the family's. You can switch the milk to 2 percent, 1 percent, or skim. Keep adding a variety of foods to his palate, but don't force foods he doesn't want or make him eat when he isn't hungry.

At this age, children enjoy routines and repetitive motions. Consequently, they may enjoy eating the same foods repeatedly or even developing their own rituals (such as wanting to eat the same meals every day). Some will be adventurous and try whatever you put on their plate. Others will stick to what they like. Provide toddlers with between-meal snacks at regular times and endeavor to make those snacks nutritious! Little stomachs

WARNING

Just because they can now run, jump, and talk, this age of child is still in danger of choking on many ordinary foods. It is still wise to cut up grapes, hot dogs, and apples for this age group. Avoid nuts and popcorn as well as they can become lodged in the throat.

empty fast and need to be refueled. Also keep in mind that kids this age love candy and sweets, but these should be kept to a minimum and definitely out of sight.

Though it is tempting to use food as a reward, especially when potty training, it is best to use praise for a reward. Moms and dads who clap and get excited about their children's progressive toilet training can be just as effective as the parent who uses candy. Praise compliant and appropriate behavior, and every time you see good eating habits beginning to form, praise your child for their behavior.

It also helps to give children this age a choice between two types of foods when they are fussing about what to eat. For example, say, "You can have tuna or peanut butter on your sandwich. Which do you want?" This way you have control over the choices, and the child feels in control of making the choice.

The Preschool Years

In general, four-year-olds weigh between twenty-seven and fifty pounds and are thirty-seven to forty-six inches tall.[11] Height variations are common in children this age. Usually this is due to other measures, such as genetic factors, nutrition, the environment, and their overall health.

Most kids at this age can feed themselves quite well and manipulate their cups with ease. As a child reaches the three-and-a-half year mark, he can become more demanding and less cooperative. How many of you remember how upset your child became when you cut her sandwich the "wrong" way? She wanted diagonals and you gave her horizontal halves! The nerve! Note: The trick is to react calmly to this type of battle for control and not to get into a contest of wills over a sandwich.

Though the four-year-old may not have the greatest appetite, she can eat independently, which is certainly helpful to parents. Usually the only help she'll need will be to cut up her food into smaller pieces. Some kids at this age are slow eaters or may continue to insist on the same foods and refuse specific foods, but children's appetites and willingness to try other foods seem to improve the closer to age five they become.

Even though it is difficult, parents need to remain as relaxed as possible when it comes to mealtimes. Present a variety of nutritious foods and keep your approach low-key. If a child this age senses that eating really matters to parents, he may try to engage you in a power struggle over the food, portions, or mealtime in general. Therefore, present the meal, praise good eating habits, and encourage your child to try a variety of foods, even if it means only trying one spoonful.

At this age, kids need to eat five times a day—three meals and two snacks. Snacks should be given early enough that they don't interfere with scheduled mealtimes. A good plan is to have your child finish a snack at least an hour before he eats. This way he won't ruin his appetite with the snack. By age four, kids should eat foods the family eats. At every meal, preschoolers should be asked to take one bite of a food even if they don't think they will like it. Keep in mind, all other family members need to model this example for it to work effectively. If your teenager studies his plate and announces to the rest of the family, "This casserole is so gross," your five-year-old will almost certainly model that behavior.

> **EVEN THOUGH IT'S DIFFICULT, PARENTS NEED TO REMAIN AS RELAXED AS POSSIBLE WHEN IT COMES TO MEALTIMES.**

If your child doesn't like what has been prepared, don't make another meal just for him. Instead, you can wrap up the uneaten food and offer it again when he is hungry (which will likely be about an hour later). If you begin offering alternative meals, you teach your child to be a picky eater. (You should get used to being a short-order cook as well if you do this.) Some kids grow out of this stage of picky eating; others don't. If your child is a picky eater and refuses certain foods at mealtimes, you must retrain him to eat healthy.

Here is what Dr. Kolp-Jurss suggests: Pick a stress-free time of a day and tell your child that she is expected to eat what everyone else in the family eats. There will be no more special meals or no alternative meals prepared. Then make sure you have very little junk food in the house and refocus your child on healthy eating. Keep presenting the meals. It may take twenty meals (or some other number) until your child will begin to engage with the family.[12] Yes, you read that right—which means you really have to persist with this strategy. You can't give up after ten or twelve tries if you see no improvement. Hang in there until you notice a change.

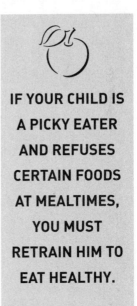

IF YOUR CHILD IS A PICKY EATER AND REFUSES CERTAIN FOODS AT MEALTIMES, YOU MUST RETRAIN HIM TO EAT HEALTHY.

If your child refuses to eat, simply tell him that it is his choice. Then inform him when the next opportunity to eat will be. Don't make him sit at the table for hours until he cleans his plate. He won't starve by waiting for the next meal. Eventually he'll realize that when he is hungry, there are structured times to eat and that he will have to adjust to the schedule.

School-Age Kids (Ages 6-12)

Typically, school-age kids gain around five to seven pounds a year with girls having a growth spurt around age 9-10 and boys around 13-14 years of age. Parents should be aware that there is a prepubescent "plumpness" that often precedes the puberty growth spurt. While it could be true that such plumpness is part of a weight problem, it may also be that these kids are getting ready to grow into their weight as puberty is soon to come.

> **WHEN GIRLS ARE OVERWEIGHT, PUBERTY CAN START AS EARLY AS EIGHT OR NINE YEARS OF AGE.**

When girls are overweight, puberty can start as early as eight or nine years of age. Early signs for girls are developing breasts and growing hair under the arms and in the pubic area. While the average age of menstruation remains at age twelve or thirteen, more children are entering early puberty.[13] Furthermore, the number of girls reaching early puberty is much higher for African-American girls (age 9=77 percent, age 7=27 percent) than Caucasian girls (age 9=33 percent and age 7=7 percent).[14]

One of the theories as to why girls are maturing early relates to the increased fat being seen in kids today. With more body fat is an increased likelihood that a girl will begin to produce estrogen, and increased estrogen can bring on early development. There may be other factors such as exposure to certain chemicals and other environmental concerns to consider as well.

Boys this age can grow in height at a rate of around two inches a year. Their long bones (arms and legs) are lengthening and can sometimes cause growing pains. If your son complains of aching bones, take his pain seriously. He may not be making it up.

It is during the school-age years and when peer relationships develop that parents typically see the impact of having an overweight child. Low self-image can begin to develop when other kids tease and say cruel things to an overweight child. Consequently, some kids miss out on the normal social interactions needed to improve their social skills. Parents can help their child to better handle teasing and rejection, as we will see in chapter nine.

In general, eating should be its own activity, not something done on the run or when watching TV or doing something else. With school and activities, it's tempting to eat in the car or relax in front of the television with food. When you do, you are helping to instill bad habits. At this age, kids need to eat nutritiously and get enough sleep. If parents could enforce these two things, most kids would function better at school.

Enforce That Bedtime!

Sleep is so important for kids. It gives their bodies a chance to re-energize. In general, school-age children need about ten hours of sleep a night. Many don't get this and are tired and cranky as a result. Of course, every child is different and their needs may vary a bit from this number, but the important thing is to help your child get enough sleep to be rested the next day.

In terms of snacks, offer plenty of fresh fruits and vegetables. If the only snack foods in your home are junk food, kids will automatically pick those foods. Yet if you have only healthy snacks, they'll have no choice! Fruit can look rather unappealing next to the bag of highly seasoned, salty chips, but when there are no chips and fruit is the only option, it's amazing how good that fruit tastes for a snack. Our children are no different from us. When you go up to the dessert table at a buffet and the choices are decadent chocolate cake or grapes and cantaloupe, which do you pick? If you have a bunch of sweets and chips in the house, they'll want to eat them.

Ten-year-old Billy is full of energy and activity. His love for science leads him to spend hours exploring the tiny marsh behind his house. Billy finds new swamp insects and plants each day which he documents carefully using several of his fun science books. Because he's always hungry, as he runs in and out of the house to fill containers and bottles with his findings, Billy makes a point to stop a minute and grab a snack on each occasion. He usually has a snack of chips, cookies, and juice when he comes home from school too.

His mother loves his inquisitive mind and marvels at his unbounded energy. Because she wants to support his science interest, she rarely requires Billy to stop his activities and eat meals with the family. In addition, there is a new baby to care for and her attention is often pulled toward the infant and off of her older child. However, Billy's mom notices that Billy is gaining weight. Concerned, she makes an appointment with a registered dietitian.

The dietitian does a quick assessment of Billy's eating habits and notes the lack of structure and planning for after-school snacks and the dinner meal. The correction was simple: After school, Billy was to have a highly nutritious snack taken from the bottom of the Food Pyramid (several suggestions were provided). A structured dinnertime was to be established and maintained. When snack- and dinnertimes arrived, Billy was to stop playing and eat. The registered dietitian reassured his mom that Billy's science interests could be put on hold long enough to eat a nutritious snack and dinner. His brain would benefit even more from proper refueling.

These small changes made a big difference. Best of all, Billy was no longer hungry for hours on end. Though the quantity of food he was to eat increased, the number of calories he took in dropped significantly. Eating well allowed Billy to eat more and fill up—and he began to grow into his weight.

Billy's mom realized that her son still needed the structure she used to provide for him. Even though it was easier to allow Billy to pursue his love for science outdoors and take care of his own eating needs, she had misjudged Billy's growing independence when it came to feeding himself. In fact, she often wondered why Billy just picked at his food when the family did have dinner together, especially since she had heard Billy say how hungry he was the minute he walked in the door from school.

What she now realized was that Billy was like most kids his age. Left to his own choosing, he would pick the appealing high-calorie snacks that offered little nutrition over the healthier choice. Those unhealthy snacks had become the main source of his late day diet. Billy wasn't developmentally ready to be completely independent with his eating. He still needed her guidance and teaching.

While it is important to have developmental markers and be aware of specific issues that are important in feeding your child, keep in mind these are only guidelines. Every child is unique and may reach these developmental stages sooner or later. Also keep in mind that some children have food allergies or must avoid certain foods because of medical conditions.

Keep trying when it comes to feeding your family healthy food. And if you have questions about your individual child's dietary needs, contact a registered dietitian for help. Such professionals can provide great information and tailor an eating program to your child's specific needs.

POINTS TO PONDER

1. Prevention begins as early as before you conceive a child.

2. Overfeeding an infant can set that child up for a weight problem later in life.

3. Diets are not for toddlers. Doing so could restrict the nutrition they need for growth.

4. Two- and three-year-olds typically don't eat three "good" meals a day. If your child eats one healthy meal and tends to snack at other meals, your child is behaving quite normally.

5. Parents should avoid getting into power struggles over food with preschoolers.

6. It's important not to confuse prepubescent "plumpness" with being overweight. However, take action if your school-age child is overweight so that a too-early puberty is prevented.

6
Let's Move!

Ten-year-old Tim spends seven hours of his school day sitting in a fifth-grade classroom. There is no recess or PE because both have been eliminated due to budget cuts and school policies. When the final bell of the school day rings, Tim walks to the school bus and spends another thirty minutes riding home. When he and his younger brother finally arrive home around 4:00 p.m., he heads for the TV. On his way, he grabs a bowl of ice cream with a generous squirt of chocolate syrup. Then he turns on the Disney channel to watch two of his favorite television shows.

Now rested from school, he goes to his desk to do an hour's worth of homework. Soon it is time for dinner. Since everyone's schedule is different in this single-parent home, there is no family meal. Tim prepares his own dinner by heating up two pieces of frozen pizza and adding some chips to his plate. He washes his meal down with a Coke.

After dinner, Tim must practice his trumpet for the school band. When finished, he heads up to his room to play a favorite video game for an hour. Bored with the video game, Tim logs onto his computer and finds a few friends to Instant Message (IM). Pretty soon, it's time for a shower and bed.

After reading this brief account, it's easy to see why the numbers of overweight kids in our country are growing. Why? Because Tim is not unique. He represents many children from many families who simply do not get enough activity into their day to balance out what they eat. Like countless other kids, Tim has been sitting still all day, even though his day has certainly been full of mental activity. Equally concerning is the fact that Tim's diet needs some serious revision. He is consuming too many calories with too little nutrition, and because he isn't physically active, he is overweight.

The good news is Tim's lack of activity doesn't have to remain that way. His mom can provide Tim with healthier, more nutritious foods. To do so, his mom will need to rid the house of junk food and stock the refrigerator with fruits, cheeses, and whole-wheat grains in the form of bagels and English muffins. In addition, she'll have to find new ways to get Tim moving more throughout the course of his day, because he can't just cut back on food—he needs to be active to see real change.

Granted, Tim has to go to school, but Tim's mom could advocate for recess or physical education to be reinstated back into his school's curriculum. Most likely this effort would not yield immediate results, but it would be a start. There are organized methods and channels for parents to use in order to advocate such changes, as we will discuss in a later chapter.

Tim lives too far away to walk or bike to school, and his mom is not interested in changing schools. So there isn't much she can do about the number of hours her son sits during the day. However, the time after school is another matter. Though his mom works until 6:00 p.m., she can arrange for Tim and his younger brother to go to the local YMCA in the hours after school. The YMCA has a supervised physical fitness after-school program, and the cost is minimal. It's actually cheaper than paying a neighbor to supervise the boys until she gets home from work, which has been her current practice. And with his mom's written permission, the school bus will actually drop Tim and his brother off at the door to the facility. Tim's mom will then swing by the YMCA to pick up the boys on her way home from work.

When everyone arrives home, Mom could serve a nutritious dinner that was prepared over the weekend or the night before. This takes planning on her part, but the benefit is that she will have healthy meals ready to go when she walks in the door. All she has to do is heat them up in the microwave . . . and the entire family will appreciate her efforts as they are able to sit down at the table and eat together while talking about their day.

One other important change: TV should be off-limits during school days. Mom talks to Tim and both agree—no TV. After dinner, Tim's mom invites both boys to take a short walk with her. She may need to head to the neighborhood grocery store (in which case the boys can carry the groceries), or perhaps they will just take a quick lap around the neighborhood. As they walk, Tim's mom makes a game as to who can take the biggest steps and jump over the sidewalk cracks.

After the walk, Tim practices trumpet and does his homework. Mom jokingly has Tim give her ten sit-ups for every ten minutes he sits and works. They laugh and Mom joins Tim doing the sit-ups. "Tim, we can get your brain fit and our bodies fit at the same time." Then, instead of isolating in his room with media after the work is done, Tim is encouraged to play hide-and-seek with his younger brother while his mom cleans up the kitchen. This activity requires him to hustle up and down the stairs multiple times. Later, after his shower, Tim settles down for bed with a book.

These suggested changes will add up to a big change in Tim's health, yet they aren't huge to implement. Tim still spends the majority of the day sitting because of the requirements of school, the commute to and from school, and homework and band practice. Yet his family has made intentional changes to help Tim become more active. Small changes add up over time. Specifically, Tim was encouraged to run off some of his energy after sitting all day by joining an after-school YMCA program. Media was discouraged and interactive play encouraged. A family meal-time was instituted with mild exercise being required after dinner.

Research now shows that as children get older, they are less likely to be physically active.[1] This is due in part to their increased consumption of media as well as the sedentary lifestyles of their parents. The earlier you teach your children the importance of an active lifestyle, the better.

The Benefits of Being Active

Kids need to be active for a number of reasons. They are developing muscle strength, balance, coordination, and motor skills. Physical activity assists this development. In addition, their bones are growing and exercise positively influences bone development. Physical activity also improves cardiovascular health as well as overall health. According to the American Heart Association (AHA), physical exercise not only helps reduce weight, blood pressure, the risk of diabetes, and some kinds of cancer, but also improves the good cholesterol and psychological well-being in kids. Finally, activity helps prevent obesity. Inactive kids become inactive adults!

Make Time for Exercise

The AHA recommends that kids get sixty minutes of moderate to vigorous exercise every day. By "moderate" they are recommending walking fast or purposely and exerting some energy. Very young children ages two and older should have at least thirty minutes of moderately intense daily physical activity. At least three to four times a week, they should get thirty minutes of rigorous physical exercise in order to help their lung and heart fitness.[2] If you cannot find a thirty to sixty minute block of time for such activity, you can break up activity times into ten to fifteen minute blocks and complete the recommended times for healthy exercise throughout the day.

If your child does not have a physical education class or recess in her school day, you will have to make an extra effort to get her moving when she is home, which means addressing how she spends time after school, in the evenings, and on weekends.

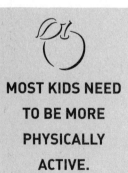

MOST KIDS NEED TO BE MORE PHYSICALLY ACTIVE.

The bottom line is this: most kids need to be more physically active. It's simply too easy to be sedentary in our culture. Children can spend days or even weeks having moved their bodies very little, and weight gain is the result. Exercise, activity, and movement have to be intentional and planned. Families need to make this happen by cultivating lifestyle changes that engage the entire family in more movement and physical activity. Small changes, such as parking the car away from the mall door and walking a longer distance, or taking the stairs instead of the elevator, or playing catch instead of watching TV, will make a difference over time.

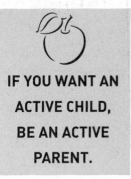

IF YOU WANT AN ACTIVE CHILD, BE AN ACTIVE PARENT.

Tater Tots and Couch Potatoes

If you are a couch potato and spend most of your free time in a state of paralysis, watching TV and with the remote glued to your hand, your kids will gradually learn to do the same—and become couch potatoes in the making! In terms of their weight, changing their activity level could make all the difference. For instance, if a hundred pound child decreased his daily television watching by one hour and instead did one hour of moderate exercise like raking leaves or riding his bike, he could lose 24 pounds in a year even if his diet didn't change![3]

If you want an active child, be an active parent. When both parents in a two-parent family exercise, their children are six times more likely to be active than children with sedentary parents.[4] Children learn lifelong habits by watching what you do. What you do, they will do. You can be a positive role model, but it means you have to get off the couch and instead take a walk, ride bikes, rollerblade, or go to the pool and swim with your kids. Take the stairs instead of the elevator, and race your children to the top! Whenever possible, walk instead of piling into the car. Yes, it will require effort, but the payoff for all of you will be worth it. And you might even have some fun.

The Importance of Play

Active play is the best way to get young kids moving. Playing is also a learning activity that encourages verbal and logical skills and the development of relationship skills. Social cooperation and leadership skills develop in children through organized play. Furthermore, we know that when parents play with their children, children have improved self-esteem and are reinforced in their imaginations and creativity.[5]

Indoor Play for All Ages

We tend to focus only on outdoor play activities, but it's important to have both indoor and outdoor play activities in mind so that when it rains, playing doesn't have to desist. An indoor play space is really important for those bad weather days in winter as well. It doesn't have to be a large space, but it should be safe and encompass a designated area. Whether you carve out a corner of a room and make it a play space or are fortunate enough to have a playroom, arrange it so that your child can jump and move around in the space.

If your child goes to day care and there are no physical areas for your child to play, you need to find a better day care facility. Those facilities that do have play areas should be safe and supervised. Your child should have at least twenty minutes of active playtime factored into his day. Play and activity are important enough that it is worth it to consider moving to a new facility.

In terms of indoor games, the possibilities are endless, but here are some suggestions to get you started. Look for the age-appropriate symbol and have fun!

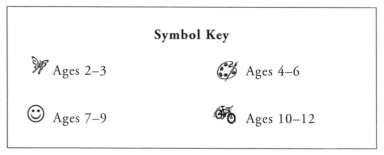

Symbol Key

🦋 Ages 2–3   🎨 Ages 4–6

☺ Ages 7–9   🚲 Ages 10–12

Dancing. Kids love to dance. Just put on the music, give them a fake microphone and a mirror, and let them do their thing. There are a number of songs that have actions to go along with the singing. You can also find a creative movement class for your three-year-old and begin dance classes as early as age four.

I volunteered in my church to do the praise and worship for the four- to five-year-olds for a few years. The songs I picked for that age group always had a lot of motion, action words, and hand gestures. Not only was I teaching them to have joy and praise God, but I was wearing them out so they could sit and listen to the teacher who did the lesson!

 Play hide-and-seek and other searching games. Hide the Thimble or a scavenger hunt are a great way to get kids moving indoors. You may have to set some boundaries as to which rooms are off-limits.

 Get a plastic hopscotch board and spread it on the floor. Another good option? Twister! (This is great fun for parents too . . . and even more fun for kids to watch their parents!)

 Bounce a balloon back and forth for a game of keep-away. Balloons do a lot less damage than rubber balls when it comes to these sorts of games, which make them safer for in the house.

Rollerblade or roller-skate in the garage. That part of the house can be a fantastic place for kids to burn off steam when the weather doesn't cooperate. All it takes is having Mom put the cars in the driveway.

Indoor bowling or other "active" play sorts of games. There are some marvelous toys on the market which are not too expensive and relatively soft/lightweight so they won't harm indoor furnishings. Check out end-of-summer clearance sales for some great blow-up toys with plastic balls, etc. that might be targeted for pool use but are equally great when used in a living room or play room.

Table tennis and foosball. These are great games for kids who are learning about team play, particularly that middle group between ages six and twelve.

Playing games that have been around forever. Follow the Leader and Simon Says are always a hit with younger kids. Preschoolers and toddlers will also enjoy singing songs with lively motions, like "London Bridges" and "Ring-Around-the-Rosy."

Play games that involve aiming. Darts is another great game for older kids. The many new styles available use much safer plastic-tipped or even magnetic darts which won't puncture walls (or kids). Any sort of "aiming" game with soft parts (like basketball hoops that affix to doors and use foam balls, etc.) are great too.

 Read a fairytale and act out the parts. For example, your child can be the big, bad wolf and you can be one of the little pigs whose house is about to be blown down. Dramatic reenactment not only encourages imagination but promotes interest in reading and books.

Your Part in Play

Play should be all about having fun. Keep in mind that young children love to show what they can do and want feedback and participation. How many times have you heard, "Look, Mom, look what I can do?" And then they proceed to dangle from the monkey bars or glide down the slide, or ride their bike. Your smile, nod, or "Wow!" goes a long way toward building their esteem and confidence.

Safety First

Activity brings up many questions about safety . . . with some being more easy to answer than others. Kids should wear helmets when riding bikes, and their activity should be supervised. Children should play in safe areas and not be exposed to faulty equipment that is in disrepair, and their play should be supervised. Some neighborhoods will have unsafe play equipment, and it's up to parents to deal with this problem. Whether they organize a plan for repairing the equipment or opt not to have their children play with it, the decision is one best left up to a supervising parent. A pass to a community recreational facility may fix such a problem. Or parents may have to hunt for a well-supervised facility or park that has working equipment and play areas. And also in regard to safety, don't forget to use ample amounts of sunscreen for skin protection when children are outside.

Outdoor Play for Children Ages 6 and Under

There are a host of fun games and activities for this age group that will increase their activity level. You are only limited by your imagination in terms of what passes for activity. Anything that has your child off the computer or away from the couch can qualify. And it's even better when you can be a part of the action.

> **CHILDREN SHOULD PLAY IN SAFE AREAS AND NOT BE EXPOSED TO FAULTY EQUIPMENT THAT IS IN DISREPAIR, AND THEIR PLAY SHOULD BE SUPERVISED.**

- *Tumbling.* There are organized tumbling centers, such as gymnastic centers, that provide tumbling and movement classes. When my kids were little, we spent hours every week at Gymboree—a national program geared toward physical play for newborns, toddlers, and preschoolers. The fun included music, art, and play—all of these activities being designed with the developmental age of children in mind. The great part was that parents participated with their children. There were giant hoops and tunnels through which to crawl, slides, and parachutes to hide under. If you can't afford an organized tumbling center or there isn't a center near you, get on the floor with a couple of mats or cushioned rugs and practice somersaults, rolls, and bends. Spot your children as they try to do cartwheels or other gymnastic-type moves.

- *Draw a Hopscotch board on your back patio or driveway.* Chalk from the dollar store will do the trick. Preschoolers will enjoy jumping the squares in this old-fashioned game with plenty of moving.

- *Play Frisbee.* All you need for this activity is a little room to run. This is great for two kids or more or even a single child and a dog, if the dog will cooperate. A boomerang is another good option—and especially a favorite of boys.

- *Jump rope.* This exercise is cheap and teaches coordination as well as providing great cardiovascular exercise. My daughter and her friends spent hours learning and singing rhymes to jump rope when they were younger. Check out the library or online for rhymes if you can't remember those from your own childhood. The rhymes add to the fun.

- *Martial arts.* These active arts promote discipline and movement.

- *T-Ball and soccer.* These are easy games for younger kids and can be organized in a neighborhood or in a park. There are also city leagues and programs through the YMCA.

- *Active games in the neighborhood.* Play Red-Light—Green-Light, Hide-and-Seek, Simon Says, Mother May I, Red Rover, Tag, and other active games that require motions and movements. Organize a game of kick-ball in the neighborhood. The options for this type of play are endless!

Ideas Galore!

If you need ideas for new games to play, or you want to check the rules for how to play a certain game, check out this amazing Website: www.gameskidsplay.net.[6] It has every game imaginable listed, as well as plenty of ideas for keeping your kids at play. Whether you need a travel game for time spent in the car, a game for the whole neighborhood, or some new jump-rope rhymes for your daughter and her friends, this website has it.

- *Biking or skating.* Put on the training wheels, helmet, and pads and teach your child to ride a bike. Take family bike rides. For skating, there are beginner skates that make learning to skate easy. With helmets, knee pads, and elbow pads, they will be more secure if they fall. Lace up your own skates, take their hands, and teach them how.

- *Take a walk.* Whether you walk the dog or go for a short walk, walking is good for you and your child. If your child can walk, get her out of the stroller and taking steps on her own. Though this can be inconvenient because toddlers walk slower due to their short legs, they need to move. It might be easier for the parents to use a stroller, but it doesn't benefit the children as much.

- *Go on outings.* Whether you go to the park, zoo, museum, or other interesting places, walk and see what there is to see. Find a safe park with good equipment and make a weekly event out of going. Meet with other moms with small children for a time of fellowship so you have an outing too. Go down the slide with small children. Let them climb the monkey bars and explore the tubes and slides.

- *Fly a kite.* This can be great fun when the weather cooperates. Let your child pick out a kite, put it together, and fly it at a nearby park or beach.

- *Explore the outdoors.* When my children were little, we loved to be little botanists. We would look at all the leaves and the different shapes, find insects, jump through puddles, and explore trails and parks. You can go on a nature hunt for items of interest.

- *Play in the snow.* If you live in a cold weather environment, dress your children in warm clothes and send them outside to make snowmen, forts, and snow angels. Introduce them to cold weather sports such as ice-skating, skiing, snowboarding, and cross-country skiing. I still remember my first pair of ice skates at age four; they had double blades to help with balance.

- *Sandbox play.* Yes, sandboxes can create quite the mess, but kids still love to play in them. Add a little water and they can sculpt fantastic creations.

Avoid competitive play with young children. At this young age, children are being introduced to physical activities that require skill building and increased coordination and balance. They should be allowed to learn at their own pace since everyone's growth and development may not be the same. You should aim to provide an opportunity to practice games and sports that require the use of gross and fine motor skills rather than pressuring children to excel at a given sport. Play is good just for the sake of play.

If your day is so overly scheduled with routine and chores that there is little in the way of fun for your child, work to remedy the problem. The key is to find activities that you and your child like and then do them regularly. Sometimes we have to put down the dust rag and pick up the tennis racquet. Even though it might not seem like it now, our children will remember the time we spend playing with them, not how clean the house was.

And don't be afraid to try new things. It's important to show your child that trying new activities can be fun even if it is a little scary. When my son wanted to learn to rollerblade, I had never done it before. But I strapped on a pair, and the two of us learned together. When he was a child, we spent hours skating together. Both of us found out that we really enjoyed this activity. I still do it to this day! And if I ask my son, he'll still go with me.

If your child is fearful of an activity, try to find out why. You may be able to allay her fears by talking about it. Then slowly expose her to different kinds of activities until she finds one she is willing to try. If, for example, she is afraid to skate, move on to something else. In time, she may be ready to try skating. Don't make fun of her for being afraid or shame her into trying something she is hesitant to do. Instead, encourage and coax a little. If you still meet resistance, drop the activity and try something different. Kids will try new activities when they are ready and feel confident based on their own timetable.

Children between ages seven and twelve will want to be in organized sports. It's wise to hold off introducing kids to competitive sports until age eight or older because of the risk for physical injury. It should be a given that children playing competitive sports have proper gear and be taught how to prevent injury. Kids this age should not be using free weights or doing weight training to prepare for a sport, because they are too young in terms of their physical development.

A child's attitude toward physical activity is so important. Some kids don't play sports because they fear failure or are easily frustrated. If either reason leads to avoiding sports, find a sport your child might like that is less competitive. Encourage him to keep trying while consistently praising his efforts and demonstrated improvement. For example, a child who feels inferior to other kids because he is small for his age might do well learning how to use golf clubs and practicing with his dad since golf is more individually focused.

Sometimes a child's attitude toward sports and games has everything to do with the parents' attitudes. If parents are critical, focused on winning, pushy, or driving their kids to exhaustion, the kids won't want to play. When the game isn't fun anymore and becomes an arena for shame and humiliation, there is nothing healthy about the physical activity. You can probably think of a time when you saw a child being shamed for his failure at sports.

KIDS WILL TRY NEW ACTIVITIES WHEN THEY ARE READY AND FEEL CONFIDENT BASED ON THEIR OWN TIMETABLE.

During one of the years my husband coached an elementary basketball team, one of the dads yelled and screamed at his son from the sidelines during practices and the games. When the boy made a mistake, he checked his dad's reaction with fear and trembling, because the anger on the dad's face was visible. It was heart-wrenching to watch. The boy's esteem dwindled as the season continued. I finally suggested that the dad let the coach do the coaching and instead keep quiet, but it didn't matter much since this man was on his child's case after each practice. Basketball held no joy for this young man, and he couldn't wait for the season to end.

The recreational soccer league in our area responded to the increasing number of parents acting out by requesting that parents sit in silence for one entire game. All we were allowed to do was clap when our kids scored a goal. The game was eerily quiet, but the point was made. If you have nothing good to say to your child in the sports arena, don't say it. The idea of the soccer league was to encourage physical activity, not make it so competitive and aggressive that kids didn't want to play. When kids feel that their esteem is on the line because of parent expectations or unrealistic standards of performance, sports can be emotionally damaging, both to the child and the parent-child relationship. You may win games if you push your child in a negative and critical way, but you'll lose his heart and destroy his spirit.

One reason parents negatively react when their child plays sports is because they are vicariously living through the experience and see their child's performance as a reflection on them. This is narcissistic and unhealthy—the activity is about you and not your child. Well, it shouldn't be. Children's sports are about encouraging your child to be active and do her best.

If you want your child to be active in a sport, ask him what sport he may want to play. Encourage exploration and try a number of different activities. Don't push a sport simply because *you* like it. When your child agrees to try a sport, if you can coach, do it. If you can't, be at his games and cheer for him. Support his efforts, praise any improvement you see, and help to build his esteem. Don't compare him to other kids and constantly point out his shortcomings, as this will only discourage his progress. Easily frustrated kids need help understanding that they will get better at the activity with practice. Few people are immediately good at a sport. Most of us have to work hard to do well at an activity. Even gifted athletes have to practice, practice, practice.

Outdoor Play for Children Ages 7–12

- *Baseball and softball.* If your child played T-ball, he may be interested in moving up to softball or baseball. Even if he didn't play T-ball, these sports can be learned and practiced with parents. Your child will remember the hours spent throwing a ball in the back yard, or the time you took to show him how to handle a bat and swing at the ball.

- *Jump rope.* This activity is suitable for kindergarten-age kids, but it's really great for older children. Jumping rope is particularly fun when there are three or more children involved. By jumping with one large rope (have two kids swinging the ends) or double-dutch jumping (swinging two ropes), the rhymes and fun just increase. This is definitely one activity parents can get into as well!

- *Swimming.* This is another activity that is great for all ages of children. Whether you swim at a community pool, country club, or fitness center, get kids into the water and they will get active.

- *In-line skating or rollerblading.* This is a fun way to be active, provided you have the pads and protective gear needed to guard against falls. Parents can skate with their kids and exercise while engaging in social time with their kids.

- *Basketball.* There are community courts and parks with hoops available. Hoops can be purchased for a driveway or neighborhood game too. Find a place to play and practice with your child. If you aren't into basketball games, consider other games such as PIG and Around-the-World.

- *Football.* This is not my choice. (Do I sound like a mom, or what?) I've seen too many kids with concussions to be a real advocate of this sport, but if your child is going to play, make sure he has the proper equipment and gear.

- *Soccer.* This game is great for running and staying fit. Though it can be a vigorous game with occasional injuries, being part of a soccer team builds comradery and cooperation into kids.

- *Wrestling, tennis, and other sports.* Many schools offer a variety of sports from which your child can choose and participate.

- *Seasonal sports.* Whether they snowboard in winter or surf in the summer, these are good activities for kids and families. If you aren't sure how to begin, try signing up your whole family for a class that teaches the basics. Also consider cross-country skiing, snowshoes, and ice-skating.

- *Golf.* For those parents who love golf, introduce your child to the game and spend time together at the driving range practicing strokes. When my son was in grade school, we lived near a golf course that offered junior golf for kids his age. The children had to take a written and practice test on the rules and etiquette of golf before they had access to the kids' clubhouse and par-three course.

  Even if you don't have access to such a place, a parent and child can go to the field and work on their shots. As noted, for kids who don't like team competition, golf is a great idea because it's all about working on improving your personal best.

- *Dancing or gymnastics.* Enroll your

EASILY FRUSTRATED KIDS NEED HELP UNDERSTANDING THAT THEY WILL GET BETTER AT THE ACTIVITY WITH PRACTICE.

child in tap, jazz, ballet, or hip-hop classes and let her enjoy dancing as part of her fitness. Or have her make her own music and dance video. If your child has an interest in gymnastics, try her in a class and see if that interest translates to something she may enjoy. She can tumble in a safe environment with proper instruction.

- *Biking or exercising with scooters.* Safety is always the concern here. Require your child to wear a helmet and follow road rules of safety. Then encourage him to bike or ride a scooter to places rather than being driven in the car.

  When my daughter joins the swim team each summer, she is able to ride her bike back and forth to swim practice with a number of her friends. I could take her in the car, but the neighborhood pool is within bike-riding distance. She wasn't allowed to ride her bike to practice until she was ten years old. And then she had rules to follow: ride on the designated path and always stay with the group. The group had to use sidewalks and follow all safety rules. We even used walkie-talkies to track her progress and keep in contact in case anyone fell or got hurt.

- *Neighborhood games.* Kids love to play games with extra friends from the neighborhood. Whether they play badminton, kick-ball, have a scavenger hunt, or even play croquet, they will be getting some great exercise. Other favorites? Hide-and-seek and tag.

- *Camping.* Kids young and old love to camp. The outdoor air, hiking, and effort that goes into setting up camp all require physical activity. If you love to camp, here's your chance to be more physically active with your children.

- *Join active organizations.* The Boy Scouts, Girls Scouts, Audubon Club, or similar organizations encourage kids to be involved in their communities while developing their character and leadership potentials. Earning badges usually involves performing some physical activity.

- *Community activities.* Involve your children in community activities such as cleaning up the bay, clearing trash out of parks, and other worthwhile causes that require them to expend physical energy while helping a larger cause. Church youth groups often have annual events targeted at helping to better the community.

- *Participate in walks or runs for charitable causes.* In many cases, children can be sponsored to walk or run a certain distance for charity. Children are generally welcome to participate in these activities.

The list of possible activities you and your children can participate in is much more expansive than I have presented here. The point is to find something that is enjoyable to you and your family. Then start making time for that activity—schedule it in. To do so will promote a healthy lifestyle of activity for your family. Take a look at this activity chart. You can see the difference just a little extra movement makes in the overall picture of a child's weight and health. Here are just a few examples:

Activity	Calories Burned Each Hour
Sitting	30
Standing	60 to 110
Walking	120–200
Watching TV	80
Mowing the lawn	300
Raking leaves	300
Shoveling snow	600

The biggest motivator for all kids is parent praise. Praise their efforts to be more active, praise the times they play, and even better, try a sport together or take them on a walk with you. Most of all, make activity fun. You *can* compete with a Game Boy because activity involves *you*. In the heart of every child is the desire to spend time with parents and be nurtured. Physical activity provides you a way to do both while making memories along the way. Let's move!

POINTS TO PONDER

1. Physical activity improves a child's health and is a key factor in preventing overweight kids.

2. Kids need thirty to sixty minutes of moderate to vigorous exercise each day. You can exercise in one block of time or break exercise up into multiple times a day.

3. Small changes in your daily routine make a big difference—take the stairs, walk, or bike instead of driving to the neighborhood store, rake the leaves yourself instead of hiring the neighbor kid, etc.

4. Plan activities for your children for both indoor and outdoor occasions; make being active a lifestyle change.

7

Motivation Is the Key

Dear Dr. Linda,

We would like our daughter Hannah to care more about what she eats. We've coaxed her, cajoled her, promised her new toys, and tried about five different fitness programs. She just doesn't seem to be motivated to do anything about her weight. As we become more and more frustrated with her, we've noticed we are arguing and yelling more. This can't be good for any of us. And she seems more withdrawn and down. We feel like we are nagging her all the time. How do you motivate a child who doesn't seem to care if she is overweight?

—Frustrated

This is a great question. Motivation is important when it comes to making changes. Hannah probably does care about being overweight, especially if the other kids notice and say things about her weight. She probably feels as frustrated as you do, and yet she doesn't know what to do. There are a number of methods to motivate our kids when it comes to changing patterns and addressing the problem of being overweight.

What Motivation Is

When we feel frustrated, it's easy to nag our kids. Even though we remember our own moms nagging us and even how much we hated it, we still manage to nag our own kids. The activity of nagging is rooted in fear—fear that a child (or spouse) either won't accomplish something or will do something that will have negative consequences. Nagging is often used as a desperate attempt to motivate, but it doesn't work . . . for the most part. If nagging does motivate, there is also a tendency for resentment to build toward the person doing the nagging.

How Motivation Works

A better strategy is to use praise. In terms of developing good eating habits and exercise, you want to praise your child every time you see him exercising or eating healthy—any behavior that will help him to achieve a healthier weight. To praise your child means to give him feedback on behavior that you want to see more often because you like it. In essence, the parent should describe the behavior that was observed and appreciated and then add a positive remark or exclamation. Praise is a positive and a powerful way to motivate children. Praise is simply a description of what your child did that you want to see more often. The sooner you praise the behavior, the better—children will then associate parental approval with making a given choice.

- Sam, you made a great choice for your snack today when you picked grapes over chips. Good job!

- Molly, I sure like how you picked up your room without being told just now. Nice work! Now we can go do something fun together since your chores are finished early.

- Alex, I'm so proud of how you chose bike riding for our family activity instead of watching a movie—you are really working on helping us all become more healthy.

Be careful to praise *behavior* not his or her overall goodness. Consider these two statements aimed at motivating five-year-old Charles to eat more green beans:

- Charles, you ate two green beans. That is really good.
- Charles, you are such a good boy for eating two green beans.

There is a small but important difference here: In the first statement, Charles is praised for the *behavior* of eating green beans—he is told that eating green beans is really good. In the second statement, Charles is told that his *goodness* depends on eating green beans. The first statement praises the behavior and tells Charles that it makes his parents really happy when he eats green beans. The second statement reassures Charles that he is in good standing for now because he ate the green beans—that by doing so he has gained Mom and Dad's approval. The message being sent is not that he needs to eat more beans, but that he needs to please his parents by going through the motions.

What Would You Do?

Suppose your ten-year-old son, Ryan, was given a puppy only after he promised he would take the new pet for a walk every day. One week into owning the dog, you are growing frustrated because your son walked the dog on the first day but has not carried out his promise since then. Early into the second week, Ryan walks the dog without being asked. Which of these responses would most closely match your own?

- "Ryan, it's about time you took the dog for a walk. When will you learn that it's important to keep your promise?"

- "Thanks for walking the dog, Ryan. I wondered when you would remember to do that since you promised and have only walked the dog once."

- "Wow, Ryan, I saw you take Bomber out for a walk. That was great and I bet Bomber enjoyed it a lot."

- No verbal response is needed since Ryan is doing what he promised to do, not something requiring praise.

The best way to praise is to use the third response because it reinforces Ryan doing what he promised to do.

Praise needs to be specific. To illustrate the point, consider this analogy: When I make meatloaf, I use hamburger and ground turkey, eggs, bread crumbs, seasonings, and ketchup on top. If I asked you what you put in your meatloaf, chances are your recipe would be different. You might use cheese, mushrooms, green pepper, or other ingredients. If we asked ten people what they put in their meatloaf, we'd get a variety of recipes, but all of us would call our food "meatloaf." The term *meatloaf*—is general and will bring a different picture or memory of how it tastes to different people.

When a parent praises a child with a general statement like "You are such a good boy," it's like saying, "Mmm, good meatloaf," at a Meatloaf Cook-off. The child won't be sure exactly what Mom saw that she liked. (And you won't know why *your* meatloaf tasted good amid fifty other varieties of the same food.) The praise is too general. What did the child do that was so good? What were the specific ingredients of the good behavior? The more specific you are in your praise, the more your child will act in appropriate ways. There will be no guessing involved in terms of what you like and expect.

You can't overdo praise either. When you are honest and authentic, children eat it up. They love to hear praise; it builds their esteem. Contrary to what some people think, you don't give a child a big head or spoil him by giving him praise for appropriate behavior.

Finally, praise is biblical. As we praise God for what He does and who He is, our spirits lift and we please our heavenly Father. The same is true when we use praise with our children. When we praise positive behavior from our kids, their spirits are lifted and they want to please us. An added bonus is that we feel better about them because we are focusing on their positive behavior. Praise should be a regular part of the parent-child relationship. Praise motivates your child to do what is right and should be the first line of offense when change is desired. Praise often with a warm and affirming voice. As your child learns to make good choices and understands the consequences of those choices, stay positive and affirming. Praise those healthy decisions, and let it be known that you've noticed.

Are Rewards Appropriate?

The question always comes up about whether it is appropriate to use rewards to motivate kids to exercise and eat well. The answer is YES, but *what* and *how* you reward is important. First and foremost, kids want their parents to notice what they are doing. Think of the many times your child has said, "Watch me!" while demonstrating a new skill. And when you follow up with praise for the watched behavior, your child loves it.

WHEN WE PRAISE POSITIVE BEHAVIOR FROM OUR KIDS, THEIR SPIRITS ARE LIFTED AND THEY WANT TO PLEASE US.

However, there are times when it takes more than praise to motivate a child. When this is the case, the first thing to do is choose one behavior to change. Be intentional about the change. For example, you might say, "We are all going to work on eating more vegetables at meals." You could simply provide a reward when your child makes a healthy choice. With the current example, you might offer the following reward: "Anyone who eats all their vegetables at dinner gets to stay up for fifteen extra minutes tonight." If staying up late is a strong motivator for your child, this reward might help him eat the vegetables he normally wouldn't want to eat.

The reward given should be something your child enjoys. If it isn't, you won't see the desired results. Young children can usually be motivated by a chart with stickers to which they add more stickers as a reward. Others need a little more. Grab bags with inexpensive toys or fun items are another good option for young kids—choosing a prize is a big deal. A hat, bag, or pillow case would all work for the grab bag. Avoid using money unless you use small amounts like pennies. You don't want to buy your child's compliance.

Parents sometimes make the mistake of using the same reward over and over. After a while, the reward loses its effectiveness because the child is tired of it or no longer finds the reward so desirable. The key is to use a variety of rewards so the child stays motivated.

The Wrong Reward

A parent wanted her son to exercise more, so she set up a chart with him in order to track his daily progress. Each day, his compliance to the exercise program was charted. The boy was told that after a month of faithful exercise, he would be rewarded with a boat. The assumption by everyone was that the boat would be a model boat, toy, or perhaps even a remote-controlled vessel. *Wrong.* After a month, it was time for the boy to receive his reward. It turned out that the mom bought her son a real, life-sized boat that was ready to sail! Understandably, this reward was way out of line. The parent offered too much for too little.

The younger your child, the more immediate a reward needs to follow the desired action. That's why hugs and kisses work well. You can give them immediately. The same is true of praise. Kids can lose motivation to change when they have to wait too long to receive a reward. For example, having a child walk the dog every day for three weeks so he gets to pick the family game for a Saturday night wouldn't work for most kids—it's too little reward for too much activity, and also too long in the coming.

Spend some time watching your child to see how he spends his free time. For example, a dad noticed that his daughter loved to listen to music and sing. He told her she could play the radio after she tried a new food at dinner. It worked! Finding rewards that work for your child requires knowing what your child likes to do. If you aren't sure what your child likes to do, simply ask. Most kids will be happy to tell you what they like or want.

The Use of Contracts to Motivate Behavior

More and more kids spend time with little or no supervision, usually because of parents' work schedules. Often kids come home from school and spend several hours in the charge of an older sibling until Mom or Dad come home. This can be a setup for overeating if there are not carefully laid-out expectations as to how the

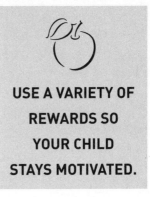

USE A VARIETY OF REWARDS SO YOUR CHILD STAYS MOTIVATED.

time will be spent. Though it is helpful to decide on rules and a schedule, a parent can go a step farther by utilizing a contract. The contract will provide accountability to do what the schedule says. A contract for children regarding time home alone should give all the information regarding how the time will be spent, what is allowed, and what the results will be if the contract is honored or not honored.

To begin, write out a clear plan for what is expected. Next, design a contract detailing the rewards and punishments that will be made if the plan is followed (see sample below). The contract will simply state what the child agrees to do and what you agree to do. Next, have everyone involved sign the contract. Finally, post the document on the refrigerator as a clear reminder to everyone that there is a contract in effect.

The plan should include answers to the following questions:

- Should a parent be called when children get home from school?

- Is media off-limits or allowed?

- What can be eaten for a snack, and when?

- When should homework be done?

- What chores need to be completed, and when?

- Is anyone allowed in or out of the house?

Each school day, ten-year-old Devon stays home with his sixteen-year-old brother after school until his mom arrives home from work. During this time, Devon has been snacking on junk food and playing video games. His mom noticed Devon is gaining weight, and she knows it isn't because of breakfast or dinner, which she cooks, or even the lunch he eats at school. His mom believes it might be a result of those hours when he is home and being supervised by his older sibling. She opts to establish a schedule and contract for the time he is out of school and until she arrives home each day.

Contracts work because they clearly state what is expected of the child and the parents and because everyone signs the contract, there is built-in accountability.

Here is a sample schedule Devon and his mom both agreed upon:

Sample Schedule

3:45–4:00	Call Mom and choose a snack (a choice of fruit, yogurt, two hard-boiled eggs, or peanut butter on whole-wheat bread)
4:00–4:15	Finish snack and change clothes
4:15–5:00	Work on homework
5:00–5:10	Set dinner table
5:10–5:30	Free time in room
5:30	Mom arrives home

The contract they wrote up looked like this:

After-School Time Contract
Name: Devon Smith
Date: January 26, 2005

My goals:

1. Follow the schedule Mom and I have agreed on.

2. Choose healthy snack when I come home from school.

3. Complete the scheduled tasks.

Consequences if I don't meet my goals:

1. Loss of video game privileges for a week.

2. Extra chores that will have to be done during my free time.

My rewards if I meet my goals:

1. Every day I follow the plan, I earn a point.

2. For every five points I earn, I get to do an activity of my choice on the weekend.

My contract will be reviewed: Every Friday night

Signed: (Mom)_____

(Devon)_____

This may seem like an overly structured schedule, but kids actually do very well with this kind of planning and structure in place. They know exactly what to expect and also what is expected of them, which means their stress is reduced and their unsupervised time is managed. In this particular instance, Devon's junk food eating and video game playing were both significantly reduced. The contract encourages him to make good choices and use his time wisely, even when his mom isn't there to supervise.

Shaping the Healthy Lifestyle

Rome wasn't built in a day, and neither is a healthy lifestyle. Change takes time and patience. While building new and positive behaviors, parents may want to use a technique called *shaping*. When you "shape" a behavior, praise is utilized for any approximation that will eventually lead to the desired behavior.

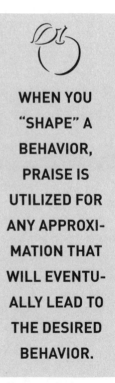

WHEN YOU "SHAPE" A BEHAVIOR, PRAISE IS UTILIZED FOR ANY APPROXIMATION THAT WILL EVENTUALLY LEAD TO THE DESIRED BEHAVIOR.

To start, decide on a goal for your child. Be specific about a behavior you want to teach. Then, break the behavior down into small steps. Finally, praise each step that takes you closer to completing the task until the goal is attained.

Suppose your three-year-old refuses to eat the cucumbers. Initially, she pushes the whole plate away when there are cucumbers as part of the meal. However, the next time you put cucumbers on her plate, she refuses to eat the cucumbers, but she does *not* push the plate away. You notice this and think, *Hey, we're getting closer to the desired behavior of trying the new food.* So you praise her by saying, "Hallie, you kept your plate by your place. Good job!"

You present the cucumbers again. This time Hallie keeps her plate by her place and even stirs the cucumbers a bit with her fork. You say, "Great job, Hallie! I like the way you stirred your cucumbers." Hallie still refuses the food, but she's getting closer to trying it, and you are determined to praise every little movement she makes toward eating it.

Several tries later, Hallie takes a bite of the cucumbers. She chews the vegetable and then spits it out, but you praise her anyway. "Wow, Hallie. You tried the cucumber. That was great!" Finally, one day, Hallie tries a bite of cucumber and swallows it. You say, "Hallie, you did such a good job eating that cucumber!" And voilá, you've just shaped your child's behavior. By praising her small approximations to try a new food, she eventually did it.

Shaping takes time because you build on behaviors until you get the one you ultimately desire. Shaping is useful when you want to teach a *new* behavior. Most of us need to be encouraged to try new things—we don't just dive into them. Some kids are more daring than others, but many need this type of intervention to send them moving in the right direction.

Motivating a Sedentary Child

I have great memories of the times my parents took me to the ice-skating rink, allowed the neighbor kids to play kick-the-can in our yard, and when they built a tree house in our old willow tree. We did many activities as a family, and I still treasure those experiences today.

Your Example

There is no way to get around the fact that parents are the most powerful role models children can ever have. The importance you place on exercise and physical activity will be reflected in the lives of your children. So if you make exercise a low priority, your family will do the same. Since exercise has nothing but positive benefits for everyone involved, make it a priority today. Get up off of that couch and start moving because it will help both you and your child.

The If-Then Contingency

Beyond following your good example, another tried and tested parenting strategy that works to motivate kids (especially older ones) to exercise is using the if-then contingency. It works like this: you take something your child really likes to do and make the opportunity to do that activity contingent upon first doing a physical activity. For example:

- If you mow the lawn, then you may play for fifteen minutes on your Game Boy.

- If you walk the dog, then you may watch that new music video you want to see.

- If you ride your bike for twenty minutes, then you may work on your model airplane.

THE IMPORTANCE YOU PLACE ON EXERCISE AND PHYSICAL ACTIVITY WILL BE REFLECTED IN THE LIVES OF YOUR CHILDREN.

Make the reward something your child really likes so he'll be motivated to do the activity and achieve the reward. Food is not to be used as a reward for exercise under any circumstances.

If this strategy doesn't work, you simply haven't found a reward that is strong enough. If you aren't sure what motivates your child, watch how she spends her free time. Whatever she does with that free time is usually an indicator of what she likes to do. I once worked with a child who loved to be by himself in his room. The reward for physical activity for him was thirty minutes alone in his room with no one bothering him. He loved the plan and it worked!

The Activities Chart

To motivate a young child, establish an activities chart and use stickers and smiley faces as rewards. Younger kids love the immediate feedback of a chart that shows their progress. You can give points for each physical activity they do and then let them trade points for stickers, pencils, erasers, and other cheap, fun items. Another option is to allow them to save up points and work toward a bigger reward. Let your children help decide what that reward will be as they will be more likely to follow through if it is something they really want.

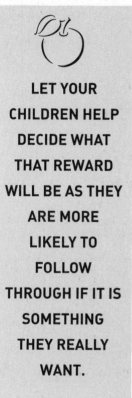

LET YOUR CHILDREN HELP DECIDE WHAT THAT REWARD WILL BE AS THEY ARE MORE LIKELY TO FOLLOW THROUGH IF IT IS SOMETHING THEY REALLY WANT.

Rewards that Work

The options are endless and only limited by you and your child's imagination, but do avoid food rewards at all costs. Some of these will work better for older or younger children, but they aren't exclusive to any particular age . . . it just depends on the child!

- Visit grandparents or a friend.

- Play catch with Dad.

- Read a story before a nap or bedtime.

- String beads.

- Do a puzzle.

- Go to the zoo or park.

- Listen to a CD or watch a music video.

- Help plant a garden.

- Color in a coloring book.

- Make an art project with colored paper, scissors, and paste.

- Take a special class, such as drawing, painting, or dance.

- Use drawing or sidewalk chalk outside.

- Sit in the "special" seat in the car.

- Blow bubbles.

- Help mom in the kitchen.

- Ride the escalator.

- Rollerblade.

- Have a friend stay the night.

- Go on a picnic.

- Choose TV show or movie to watch.

- Allow time to talk on the phone.

- Allow to stay up late.

- Camp in the backyard.

- Give extra play or "free" time.

Reward = Bribery?

Occasionally, a parent will ask if rewarding a child for making changes is bribery. Bribery concerns unethical behavior and has to do with corrupting the conduct of a person. Using rewards to motivate a behavior change is not bribery. We give grades for school work, paychecks for work completed, bonuses for special effort, and expressions of approval for a job well done. Would anyone consider these rewards to be bribery? Rewards reinforce appropriate behaviors, and since we are teaching our children to live healthier lives, these incentives help to accomplish this desire.

- Reprieve from chores.

- Play with water guns or balloons.

- Have a special time with Dad or Mom—going to a concert, etc.

Provide an Environment of Self-Regulation

Eating healthily involves a certain amount of self-regulation. For older children, this is especially necessary. There are several ways parents can promote self-regulation in children. The first is to provide clear and consistent structure and guidance. Talk to your children about why rules exist, what's behind them, and your thinking as to why healthy eating is so important. If a child understands how much you value his health, he will be more likely to internalize that value for himself and eventually change.

Guidelines and rules help motivate children to comply and also help them internalize the structure that they are expected to follow. Be clear about what you expect. A child should know what the results will be when he shows obedience and what the consequences will be when he ignores the rules.

Another help in promoting self-regulation is to give your child support for making wise decisions independently. When your child chooses a healthy snack, praise him and tell him exactly why he made a good decision. Reinforce independent positive decision-making.

TALK TO YOUR CHILDREN ABOUT WHY RULES EXIST, WHAT'S BEHIND THEM, AND YOUR THINKING AS TO WHY HEALTHY EATING IS SO IMPORTANT.

Putting It All Together

Eight-year-old Ben hates to exercise. His parents made him go to a fitness class after school in an effort to help their son. However, Ben didn't think it was any fun and doesn't want to go anymore. Now Ben's parents don't know what to do—Ben is always on the computer or playing video games. His only interest seemed to be in screens!

His parents decide to come up with a list of rewards to motivate Ben to exercise. They watch his behavior for several days and also talk with Ben about what he likes before coming up with this list:

1. Playing paintball with Dad

2. Sitting in the captain's seat of the van, away from his sister

3. Extra reading time at night

4. Extra money

5. Going to the paintball shop just to look at all the gear

6. Any gear or piece of equipment involved in paintball

7. Having a friend spend the night

8. Permission to use the Super Soakers (water guns)

9. New marbles for his collection

10. Time to play video games

Since several of these rewards involved sitting or lying down, Ben's parents opt to focus on the rewards that require more movement. As you can see from the list above, Ben likes everything about paintball. And since it is a movement activity, they recognize it could also be an opportunity for regular exercise.

Ben and his parents made up a plan. Every time his dad or mom find Ben away from a screen and doing something active like walking the dog, helping with chores, or playing outside, Ben receives a point on his paintball chart. Points can be traded in for trips to the paintball store, or they can be saved up in order to earn a reward like a paintball magazine, a piece of paintball equipment (this took lots of points but was highly motivating), or paintballs that Ben can use when he plays paintball.

In addition, Dad came up with a few war-like maneuvers Ben can use in a paintball game—these involve running, and Ben and his dad practice these maneuvers regularly. Ben's dad also challenged Ben to get some friends together to think of other "war" strategies they can practice to use in a match. Once a month, Ben's dad takes Ben and several of his friends out for a paintball game.

This plan worked so much better than an exercise class. Ben loves paintball and desires time spent with his dad, and putting the two things together turned into a perfect reward. He was highly motivated to avoid playing computer games.

After a few months of focusing on paintball, his dad asks if Ben is interested in learning golf as well. Since Ben is, the two start spending their free evenings on the driving range teaching Ben to swing a club. Ben really likes golf because it isn't so competitive. He learns the game and practices hitting balls in the backyard. Since his mom also plays golf, it is a natural choice to teach Ben's sister how to golf too. Now the family has a new activity they can all do together. When they play, they walk the course instead of using a cart in order to make the most of the game.

POINTS TO PONDER

1. Praise is the most powerful motivator for any child, regardless of the child's age or temperament.

2. Other ways to motivate children include modeling good behavior to them, using the if-then contingency, and by using rewards as an incentive for changed behavior.

3. Contracts work well for older children who are ready for more responsibility regarding how they use their time.

4. Self-regulation is important in teaching our children to make good decisions which will affect them positively and also please their parents.

8
Emotional Feeding Equals Overweight Kids

"Kim, do you want to tell me about all the candy bar wrappers your mom found under the bed?"

"I can't believe she found them. I hid them so she wouldn't know I was taking candy out of the pantry."

"Your mom isn't mad at you because you took the candy. She's more concerned about why *you are taking it to your room and hiding it under the bed. Can you tell me about that?"*

"Well, when I hide it, I have it when I need it."

"When do you need it?"

"At night, it just makes me feel better to have it in my room and know I can get it when I need it."

"Why do you need candy at night in your room? Are you feeling bad about something specific at night?"

"That's when my mom and dad fight. They don't think I can hear them, but I can. I think my dad is going to move out soon. I thought I heard him say that to my mom. I heard him say a lot of mean things to my mom, and she said mean things back. I hate it when they fight."

"So when they fight at night, how does having the candy under your bed help?"

"It makes me feel better when I eat it. It kind of calms me down, you know? It just makes me feel good. My dad brings it home all the time. So I just eat it to feel better."

"Does it make you feel better?"

"Yes, for a little while. But when the candy is gone, they're still fighting."

"So when you're upset about your mom and dad fighting, you eat candy to help yourself feel better. Is that right?"

"I guess so. I never really thought about it."

Ten-year-old Kim is using food to cope with the marital tension in her home. She feels helpless and doesn't know what to do when her parents fight. No one is talking to her about the tension she feels . . . she worries her dad will move out of the house. Every night she secretly binges on candy. Purely by accident, her mom found the wrappers stashed under Kim's mattress.

Kim's mom was reluctant to talk to her daughter about the impending divorce. She didn't want to upset Kim and thought she could keep her marital problems a secret until she and her husband made a final decision.

But Kim has sensed the tension and turned to food for comfort. In fact, Kim thinks if she even asks her mom about the fighting she hears each night, she might *cause* a divorce. No one is talking, and Kim is trying not to worry, but she still feels anxious. Food is quickly becoming her friend—or more precisely, an ally that helps her feel better for the moment. Right now, food is dependable and available to help her alleviate fear, unlike her parents. Eating candy provides this young girl with a needed escape.

> **FOOD IS QUICKLY BECOMING HER FRIEND—OR MORE PRECISELY, AN ALLY THAT HELPS HER FEEL BETTER FOR THE MOMENT.**

Kim is like a lot of kids who learn to use food to cope with bad feelings. Kids who don't know how to express their feelings or feel afraid to talk about negative feelings are especially vulnerable to using food to soothe or calm them down. When children are stressed or worried, they need to know that turning to food is not a solution and will in fact create more problems.

Emotional eating is a learned behavior developed in response to stress, negative situations, or feelings. In order to prevent emotional eating, families must reduce stress and teach their children alternative coping methods that do not use food. Children who are emotional eaters can be helped, but they must learn new strategies to handle stress.

When Stressed Means "Desserts"

STRESSED is DESSERTS spelled backwards! Perhaps this coincidence should remind us how easy it is to eat when we feel stressed. Grab a candy bar, dive into that gooey cinnamon roll, pull out the ice cream carton . . . and indulge! When you do, the stress is gone and all you feel is pleasure—for that moment. Long-term, this is not an acceptable coping mechanism because it results in overweight kids and adults. To eat to find relief for that single moment teaches us to eat when we feel stressed. Instead, we have to learn how to manage stress, eliminate it when possible, and react to it with the truth of God's Word. All of us must deal with stress; it is and will be a part of our lives. Yet we don't have to be defeated!

Stress is one of the main reasons people overeat, and stress has increased in families over recent decades. Families face all sorts of challenges—job loss and relocation related to the economy, poverty, discrimination, divorce and separation, loss of emotional support because nuclear families no longer live near extended families. If you couldn't relate to any of those stress factors, consider these: rising rates of family violence, addictions, neglect, the burden of elderly care along with care of children, longer work hours, rapid technology changes . . . the list seems endless.

WE HAVE TO LEARN HOW TO MANAGE STRESS, ELIMINATE IT WHEN POSSIBLE, AND REACT TO IT WITH THE TRUTH OF GOD'S WORD.

Children can feel pressure to perform academically, to deal with peer pressure and bullies, to adjust to changes in family living arrangements and visitation. Our children also feel great fear—of being away from home, of punishment from a teacher, of wetting themselves, of being chosen last on a team, of serious illness, of parents being called to war, of teasing and rejection from their peers. And when we factor in the tremendous pressures kids feel because they are constantly surrounded by materialism and consumerism, it's no wonder many children suffer from poor body image, eating disorders, and being overweight.

Children model their parents when it comes to stress. Translation: When you see stressed-out parents, you tend to see anxious kids. And those children often turn to food to relax and escape.

When stress hits, kids worry. Researchers Silverman, LaGreca, and Wasserstein decided to study the normal worries of schoolchildren between the ages of seven and twelve years.[1] They interviewed 273 schoolchildren and asked them about fourteen areas of worry. Here's what they found:

- The average number of worries per child was 7.64 and covered a wide range of topics, but most worried about health, school, and personal harm.

- The most frequent worries were about family, classmates, and friends.

- The most intense worries were about war, money, and disasters.

- Children's worries were related to feeling anxiety.

Another community study had researchers interview 194 children in grades 4–8 to record their worries and risk perceptions about health and the environment.[2] These kids identified concerns about personal issues, such as grades, social relations, and death, as well as more social issues such as homelessness and the environment.

Children worry because unfortunately, many have reason to worry.

Take a look at the statistics and that fact becomes very apparent. Kids are anxious because the problems and stress aren't products of their imagination at all:

- Not all kids are safe. Roughly 903,000 children (12.4 out of 1,000 children) were victims of abuse or neglect in 2001.[3]

- Many kids live with one parent who has no one else committed to share responsibilities or help with finances. According to research dating from 1999, single parents make up 27 percent of family households with children under 18.[4] Furthermore, one in two children will live in a single-parent family at some point during their childhood.[5] Most children in this situation live with a single mother. However, the proportion of children living with single fathers doubled from 2 percent in 1980 to 4 percent in 1999.[6] Another telling statistic is the fact that nearly one-third of children in the U.S. are born to unmarried parents.[7]

- Many kids experience marital tension. More than one million children have parents who separate or divorce each year.[8] Given that statistic, it isn't hard to see that as a result of the separations and divorces, many kids face new and changing family arrangements. More than half of Americans today have been, are, or will be in one or more stepfamily situations.[9]

- Many kids witness and are victims of family abuse. In a national survey of more than 6,000 American families, 50 percent of the men who frequently assaulted their wives also frequently abused their children.[10] Studies suggest that between 3.3 and 10 million children witness some form of domestic violence annually.[11]

- More and more young children are being left alone or being put into day care programs. According to the U.S. census, nearly one out of five children between the ages of five and fourteen regularly care for themselves.[12] And according to a 1997 study of families with working mothers, 41 percent of children under five years of age spend thirty-five or more hours a week in non-parental care. In 1999, 54 percent of children from birth through third grade received some form of child care on a regular basis from persons other than their parents, up from 51 percent in 1995.[13]

- Many children live in households that have housing problems, such as physically inadequate housing, crowded housing, or housing that presents a high cost burden. The percentage of households with children experiencing these problems is at 36 percent.[14]

But here's the real kicker. When kids are asked what thing they would like to change the *most* in their lives, the most frequent answer given is to have parents who are less stressed and tired. In fact, a national poll of children's concerns found that kids ages 9–14 said they only spent about 32 percent of their time with their parents because of their parents' work schedules and their own schedules.[15] And teenagers sampled in another national poll rated not having enough time with their parents and educational worries as their top concerns.[16] Kids want and need their parents! There simply is no substitute for the attention of Mom and Dad.

WHEN KIDS ARE ASKED WHAT THING THEY WOULD LIKE TO CHANGE THE MOST IN THEIR LIVES, THE MOST FREQUENT ANSWER GIVEN IS TO HAVE PARENTS WHO ARE LESS STRESSED.

Stressing the Point

Overall, the American family is more stressed but spending less time talking to each other, eating together, and vacationing together. The number of religious activities in which children are involved is decreasing, while the amount of time children spend in structured sports, passive spectator leisure activities, like watching a brother or sister play a sport, and studying (almost a 50 percent increase!), is increasing.[17]

Kids are spending less time in activities that lead to intimate family relationships and activities that equip them to handle life's problems. They spend more time in activities in which they act alone or with other kids. No wonder so many of our children feel alienated and unequipped to handle stress! Parents can help children make sense out of their stressful world and reassure them that they are safe and protected.

According to British researchers, when kids are stressed they eat twice as much at meals and snack than kids who are less stressed. In addition, they favor fatty foods and stay away from healthy options.[18] To help children combat this reality, parents must create a family-friendly home where children can slow down, relax, and not become emotional eaters.

Children learn by example, which means we parents need to relax too. Stressed-out parents create stressed-out kids. If you use food to calm or soothe yourself, your children will pick up on this as a way to cope. Consequently, you may need to work on improving your reactions to stress. Whatever eating habits you want to see in them, you need to be modeling, which means that you can't eat healthy in general yet gorge on a bag of chips when you are upset.

Sometimes we overreact. Sometimes we experience health difficulties. Sometimes financial trials bring us down. The ways we experience stress are many, yet we cannot allow that picture to be the final say. Getting rid of the stress completely may be impossible, but managing the stress well is certainly an option. Seriously consider the fifteen options here and try to implement those in your power.

1. *Recognize the stress you are under. Then remove or eliminate whatever stress you can.* Make a list of all the things that place stress on your family and then decide if any item on that list can be eliminated (see the chart at the end of this chapter). For example, if your child has too many activities scheduled and no time to play outside, which activities could be

dropped? If your current day care is causing your child problems, can you find a new day care or care arrangement? How about your own list of activities? Can you drop any extraneous meetings or commitments and spend more time with your child instead?

2. *Know the signs of stress in children.* Be able to identify the signs of an overstressed child so you can then turn to helping the child alleviate the stress. Usually the following symptoms involve a change from the normal pattern:

- sleep problems
- increased talk about bad things happening
- hyper alertness
- avoidance of events or people related to the stressful situation
- regressive behavior like thumb-sucking
- an increase in clingy and dependent behavior

- withdrawal and isolation
- restlessness
- inability to focus
- increased aggression
- blaming problems on others
- physical symptoms such as bedwetting, headaches, nausea, stomachaches, nightmares

- school failure or problems
- appetite changes

- teasing siblings or peers
- losing temper, crying

If you notice these signs in your child, don't wait. Identify those stresses that are affecting your child, and eliminate the ones you can. You may want to get family counseling to help your family deal more effectively with stress.

3. *Create an atmosphere of openness and acceptance in your home.* Stress diminishes when kids know they can talk about anything and you won't get mad or be upset. Talk with them often and encourage them to share

The Stress of Day Care

Children experience stress in poor child care environments. A child's physical responses to long-lasting stress can negatively affect development. Chronic stress produces certain hormones that can become problematic if they linger in the body. Here's what happens. When a child wakes up in the morning, there is an elevation of cortisol levels in the brain. This elevation is like a jump start to get the child up and functioning. Under normal conditions, cortisol levels fall during the morning and afternoon hours.

Children in substandard child care have a different physical experience than those in high quality care.[19] Studies show that cortisol levels remained high and actually increased for children in poor quality care. These children become more aggressive and exercise less self-control. In contrast, children in high quality care environments showed the normal decline in cortisol levels.

As you consider your child's day care facility, look for cues as to whether your child is in a stress-inducing situation. Ask yourself:

- Is there warmth among the workers? Or do they seem insensitive to the needs of the children?

- Is the staff turnover frequent? Does my child have to constantly be adjusting to new people?

- What is the ratio of staff to children? Should it be lower than it is?

- Are the workers trained in child development, and do they take seriously my child's needs throughout the day?

- Is the physical setting bright and cheery? Would I want to spend significant amounts of time here?

- When I drop by unannounced, are there factors that I see that cause me concern? Or does my child seem relaxed and happy and secure with her surroundings?

their thoughts and feelings on a regular basis. That way, when stress hits hard, they will be more likely to talk to you about how they feel and what they should do. Children who don't express their feelings or are afraid to do so are more at risk to become overeaters.

4. *Seek out support.* Parents often feel alone and overwhelmed by the stress they are under. When stress hits, it can be hard to recognize that other people have traveled the same road. Seek out friends and family who will pray with you, offer support, and encourage you through the difficult times.

Social support is a buffer for stress. Being a member of a church opens up some wonderful options that are in place to help parents just like you and me find the support we need. If your church has child-friendly programs like Mother's Day Out, go and give yourself a break from parenting for a few hours. Look for mentoring opportunities for your child in the community or at church. If applicable, attend a support group that helps with specific issues like divorce or dealing with abuse. Join a prayer group and/or Bible study and share your concerns. Allow others to pray with you and receive the support offered. Establish a relationship with a trusted friend with whom you can exchange babysitting. Any or all of these ideas will act to buffer stress in your life.

5. *Do what you can to minimize change; build routines and structure.* Children become unsettled when something out of the ordinary happens. Change is stressful, even when the change is positive. Children thrive when they are given structure and consistency—they like routine. Strive to provide structured mealtimes, bedtimes, and rules for behavior. Let your children know what is expected of them. The more predictable you are in terms of how you live, eat, work, and parent, the better they will do. And when a serious or prolonged time of stress occurs (because it happens), try to keep your routines going.

6. *Pay attention to how you are coping.* Don't ignore your own mental health. If you fall apart under stress, your children will become anxious and fearful. You communicate with your nonverbal language as well as

what you say and do. Children often sense tension and can pick up on nonverbal cues. Your well-being is extremely important for the health of your child, so you must take care of yourself. Get rest, eat right, and try to exercise.

7. *Do not overburden your children with too much.* Make your discussions of stress and problems age appropriate. Ask your children to share their questions and fears, and do your best to alleviate their concern. Reassure them of what they need to know, that you love them, God loves them, and that nothing they are doing is causing the stress.

Don't share all your problems with your children, and don't put them in the position to be a pseudo parent. If you need someone to talk to because you are struggling with your own feelings during a stressful time, find another adult or a counselor and let that person help you. *Children should not be used as sounding boards.* Going through a divorce or being a single parent can make this tempting to do, but it will only hurt your child and the relationship you have with your child.

8. *Don't avoid talking about trauma or stress.* When kids are exposed to trauma or ongoing stress, find out how they are coping. Denial or avoidance are not good methods of coping.

When there is family stress, you can help by patiently listening and being able to tolerate your children's feelings. Acknowledge their concerns and show them healthy ways to cope with the situation. Help them problem-solve. Talk about what is happening using words they can understand, and be sensitive to the fact that their reactions may differ from yours.

TALK ABOUT WHAT IS HAPPENING USING WORDS THEY CAN UNDERSTAND, AND BE SENSITIVE TO THE FACT THAT THEIR REACTIONS MAY DIFFER FROM YOURS.

Provide the hope God gives each of us to deal with difficulty—tell and show your children that you can face any circumstance or problem because God is with you. Reassure them that God will work in the situation for their good—this promise is for all who trust and believe in God.

9. *If you are married, strengthen your marriage.* One of the best ways to de-stress a family is to keep the marital covenant strong and healthy. If you need help with this, go to a marriage counselor and work on your marriage. Don't wait for the marriage to fall apart.

When we compare healthy and unhealthy marriages, we find that kids from a strong and healthy marriage are:[20]

- More likely to attend college and succeed academically
- Physically and emotionally healthier
- Less likely to attempt or commit suicide
- Demonstrating less behavioral problems in school
- Less likely to be a victim of physical or sexual abuse
- Less likely to abuse drugs or alcohol
- Less likely to commit delinquent behaviors
- In a better relationship with their mothers and fathers
- Less likely to divorce when they get married
- Less likely to be sexually active as teenagers or to contract STDs
- Less likely to become pregnant as a teenager, or to impregnate someone
- Less likely to be raised in poverty

10. *Equip your children with scriptures that speak to their fear and God's love.* The Bible has answers for how to handle problems of stress and worry. Know those answers and explain them to your children. Then help them

practice replacing their fears with the promises God gives His children by reading and praying together over these passages and prayers:

"For God has not given us a spirit of fear, but of power and of love and of a sound mind" (2 Timothy 1:7 NKJV). Prayer: *(Insert your child's name here), you have been given a sound mind because of God's spirit in you. The spirit of fear must leave as God's spirit lives inside you. I declare peace in your mind. Right now, we take every fearful thought and stop it. God, Your love takes the place of fear. Please replace any fearful thought with Your truth. We ask for peace right now.*

"Be strong and courageous. Do not be afraid or terrified because of them, for the LORD your God goes with you; he will never leave you nor forsake you" (Deuteronomy 31:6). Prayer: *Thanks, God, for being with us all the time, even when things are bad. You stay with us and get us through the problem, so we don't have to be afraid. We are never alone. We can call your name and You hear us. You are Emmanuel—God with us!*

"Therefore do not worry about tomorrow, for tomorrow will worry about itself. Each day has enough trouble of its own" (Matthew 6:34). Let's take every worry right now and tell God. Prayer: *God, we don't want to worry anymore and since You already know what will happen, we give our worry to You. You have our lives in your hand. We trust you to take care of us.*

"Do not be anxious about anything, but in everything, by prayer and petition, with thanksgiving, present your requests to God. And the peace of God, which transcends all understanding, will guard your hearts and your minds in Christ Jesus" (Philippians 4:6–7). Prayer: *Here is our request (insert request). Thank You for all You have already done and for the answer we don't see yet. Please take our thoughts and help us to think on the good things You do (list His many blessings). We know it is Your heart and desire to bless us as we live for You.*

PRAYER WORKS!

The stronger your walk with God, the more peace you will have in your home. Make time for prayer both individually and as a family. Make it a daily habit to pray *with* your children and *over* your children. If a father lives in the house, the importance of the father's blessing cannot be overstated. Every night, my husband blesses our two children at the end of our prayer time together. It is powerful. Our kids approach sleep with a sense of peace and blessing. Here is a sample of what he might say:

I bless you in the name of the Father, the Son, and the Holy Spirit with the love of God, the Peace and rest of Christ, and the joy of the Lord. May all of God's purposes be accomplished in your lives. May you grow up strong and mighty in the Lord, assured of who you are in Him, and ready to prosper in all He has for you. May your bodies be healthy and strong, your minds fixed on Him, and your emotions steady, always filled with love and kindness toward others.

11. *Encourage creative expressions of feeling though music, art, and dance.* Some kids just aren't good at putting their feelings into words. Encourage your child to express her feelings in other appropriate ways. Put on music and let her move and act out a feeling. Encourage her to draw—often you will see her worries in a picture. Then you can talk about the picture and use it to discuss her feelings. The important thing is to find an outlet that opens your child up to more expression.

12. *Limit exposure to trauma.* Exposure to violence through graphic images in media or first-hand exposure to trauma can cause stress and psychological damage. For example, if you have a spouse who is physically abusive, you and your children should not be exposed to his/her abuse. This means you may have to ask that spouse to leave or go to a shelter. Or if your child watches the nightly news with you and you notice she is more fearful at bedtime, don't allow her to see the news. Many kids would be less stressed if their parents were more discerning

about the movies and media they watch. Most of it is too frightening for kids and can cause nightmares and worries.

13. *Be physically affectionate with your children.* Touch is reassuring and makes children feel connected. Hug them, kiss them, and wrap your arms around them. Make time to sit and hold small children while you stroke their hair or cheek. Appropriate touch is healing and soothing.

14. *In the middle of a trial, talk about the good things that may come out of it and all the people who are supportive.* We can't always stop bad things from happening, yet sometimes horrible circumstances allow us to see the good in other people. For example, during a time of crisis or high stress, point out caring people who have come to your aid. Talk about how difficulty often helps us remember to depend on God and to develop patience.

God Works Through Our Difficulties

Right now there is an eleven-year-old girl in our church who needs a double lung transplant. Hopefully by the time this book is printed, Emily will have received this much-needed operation. Her family has health insurance yet had to raise an additional half a million dollars for the transplant.

Many people developed fund-raising activities to help little Emily raise the money for the transplant. One such activity involved placing donation jars by the cash register at several restaurants. When people paid for their meals, they could donate their change for Emily's transplant. One night, a man stole one of the jars from a restaurant. Understandably, people in our community could hardly believe that someone would steal a little girl's money for a life-sustaining operation. The story made the local news . . . then the national news. As a result, more people were made aware of Emily's need and participated in helping her financially. God used the bad thing someone did to bring national visibility to Emily's need.

15. *Keep children physically active as a way to release stress.* We talked about the importance of physical activity in the last chapter, but we didn't talk about how important it is for stress reduction. Physical activity helps everyone feel better when under stress. Make time for physical activity—and make the most of it by making it a family activity. Take a bike ride with your kids, go in-line skating, or walk around the block. Engage in family projects that are active, such as yard work, painting, and spring cleaning.

Behavior Problems Linked to Obesity

If your child is antisocial, anxious, dependent, depressed, headstrong, hyperactive, or withdrawn, his risk of becoming obese is potentially increased. A new study found that behavior problems might cause some kids to become overweight.[21] See a counselor and work on these problems.

It is important to intervene early in a child's life so that emotional eating can be prevented and children can learn healthy ways to cope with life. For example, a child with ADHD needs to be taught problem-solving skills in order to react less impulsively. A withdrawn child may need to be taught assertiveness skills. An antisocial child needs help with appropriate peer interactions. Role-playing can be used as a method to teach those skills. A parent with a headstrong child may have to be instructed how to hold a firm line and not give in to tantrums or other negative attention-getting behaviors.

Ignoring behavior problems makes them more difficult to change as children get older. If kids act out or are withdrawn, they risk using food in an unhealthy way. It is up to parents to notice these tendencies and seek the appropriate help.

A helpful tool to eliminate family stress is to begin a chart that first identifies that stress and then decide whether each one can be eliminated (see below). Eliminate those stressors that you can and work on the ones that can't be eliminated using the ideas we just discussed.

Family Stress	Can It Be Eliminated?
List items	*Yes or No*
Too many activities	YES
Elderly care	NO
Child being bullied	YES

POINTS TO PONDER

1. Children will often overeat in response to emotional issues.

2. Kids need adult help to unlearn emotional eating habits and replace them instead with better ways to handle stress and worry.

3. Eliminate as much family stress as possible using the fifteen strategies provided.

4. If your child has behavior problems and is eating in response to them, enlist the help of a mental health care provider.

9

Sticks and Stones . . .
Words and Hurts

Ruby was a sensitive, sweet child, always polite and never any trouble. She lived with her grandmother, Rose. One day a neighbor knocked on Rose's door and said, "You know I love Ruby like my own daughter. When she comes over to play with Angie, they have such a great time.

"The other day, I heard the girls talk about how much Ruby gets teased at school because of her weight. Ruby was crying when she talked to Angie. Anyway, here's what I wanted to tell you. I have this candy jar I keep out on a table near the door. Whenever Ruby comes over, she asks me if she can have a piece. Of course I tell her she can—that's why it is out.

"When I'm working in the kitchen, I can see the candy dish, and I notice that whenever Ruby is over, most of the candy is gone. Mind you, I don't care about the candy. Anyway, Ruby doesn't know I can see the candy jar. She walks past the candy dish many times when she is playing, sneaks a couple of pieces, and stuffs them in her pocket. She thinks no one sees her. By the time she leaves, the candy dish is almost emptied. I haven't said anything to her because I didn't want to upset her.

(Cont'd)

"I thought I should tell you this because I'm concerned about why she thinks she has to sneak and hide candy. When I asked Angie about the candy, she said Ruby's been sneaking candy for months. Apparently she has a huge box of it hidden under her bed. I just thought you should know."

Now the pieces of the puzzle were coming together for Rose. Ruby didn't talk much about being overweight, but Rose could tell it bothered her. She had spent weeks monitoring what Ruby was eating for breakfast and dinner, and even quizzed Ruby about meals at school, yet she remained unsure of why Ruby was still gaining weight. After hearing her neighbor's report, Rose decided to check under Ruby's bed. Sure enough, she found a big box stuffed with all kinds of goodies and snacks. At night, Ruby was eating in her room, alone, and gaining weight.

That evening, Grandma took Ruby by the hand and led her into the girl's bedroom. She leaned down and pulled out the big box. "Child, tell me why this is here. You don't need to hide food from your grandma. If you're hungry, I can make you a snack."

"Grandma, the kids tease me all the time and say I'm fat, so I've been trying to diet. I don't eat anything all day. I'm really good at school. But at night I am so hungry. You make a good dinner, but I am still hungry after I eat. So I have all this candy and stuff for when I get hungry at night. I can't seem to stop, and I don't want to be made fun of anymore. I didn't mean to hide the food. I just didn't know what to do. Can you help me, please?"

Ruby was struggling. She didn't know how to stop the teasing and didn't know what to do about her weight gain. The shame she felt from being teased led her to try a drastic strategy—restricting all eating at school. Obviously, this strategy wasn't working. When Ruby starved herself all day, she was hungry at night and binged on snacks and junk food. She was too embarrassed to tell her grandmother the truth and couldn't help the feeling that she was out of control.

Overweight kids like Ruby feel the brunt of teasing but don't know how to react to it. And they certainly don't know what to do to stop gaining weight. For that, they need the help of sensible parents and other adults. They need to learn how to successfully deal with both weight gain and teasing.

We Need to See the Bigger Picture

We parents and family members don't like to see our kids struggle even when we know such pain may build their character. I remember sitting in the fourth-grade classroom with one of my children's teachers. I was crying I was so upset—my child was being mercilessly teased for being the new kid in a school that rarely enrolled new kids. The teacher, a wonderful, godly woman, calmly reminded me that more was operating in this difficulty than what my physical eyes could see. I needed to focus on what *could* be done. Did I believe God was working on our behalf? Couldn't we come up with a plan to help my child?

As we prayed and trusted God for wisdom, I began to see that God was using this difficult time to develop a deeper sensitivity in this child. God was preparing his heart for an extra measure of kindness, compassion, and empathy—traits we see operating in his peer relationships today. In addition, God was teaching me not to be overwhelmed by circumstances and to trust Him.

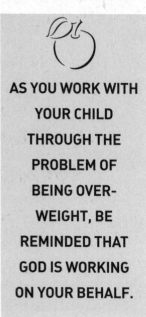

AS YOU WORK WITH YOUR CHILD THROUGH THE PROBLEM OF BEING OVER-WEIGHT, BE REMINDED THAT GOD IS WORKING ON YOUR BEHALF.

As you work with your child through the problem of being overweight, be reminded that God is working on your behalf. Struggles do build character if we respond the right way, and difficulty often leads to a deeper sense of compassion in us. Every difficulty is a training lab, an opportunity for us to teach and put into action the power of God working in our lives.

We want our kids to live in a trouble-free world, but that's not realistic. Instead, we have to teach our kids how to contend with the world, to live in it but not be driven by it, to make good choices, and to be responsible and productive, not only for the community in which we live but also for the bigger eternal purpose for which we were all created. We must also teach our children a proper foundation from which to deal with any life problem. They must know their true identity and learn to resist temptation and overcome difficulty. They don't have to live a defeated life. There is hope.

Self-control

All parents hope their children will develop the self-control needed to control overeating. Proverbs 16:32 says, "Moderation is better than muscle, self-control better than political power" (MSG). This proverb speaks to the importance of self-control in all areas of our lives. It reminds us that losing control may cost us what we want or need.

Self-control isn't some form of willpower we muster up whenever we feel desperate. God's Spirit working in us produces character traits that are found in the nature of Christ. If we want to have self-control, we must be in relationship with Christ—knowing, loving, and imitating Him. As we love God with all our heart, self-control emerges as a fruit of His Spirit operating in us. Trying to develop self-control without God's help requires self-effort and often ends in defeat. But His Spirit working in us can do amazing things. As we submit our lives to Christ, His Spirit works to develop those character traits we dearly want to see—patience, kindness, peace, goodness, faithfulness, gentleness, joy, love, and self-control.

So how do we teach our children self-control when it comes to food and eating? As parents, our job is much greater than teaching our children to exercise self-restraint when it comes to eating. We want our children to learn a broader lesson—to love the Lord their God with all their hearts, minds, and souls. We love because God first loved us. Out of that love, we desire to keep His commandments and laws. We teach them to submit their lives to Christ, to obey God, to imitate Jesus in all they do or say. As they do this, the Holy Spirit will guide them and help them develop self-control in all areas of their lives, including food and their emotions. And when we teach our children these lessons, we help them to reap the benefits of God's kingdom—one of which is the benefit of self-control.

In 2 Kings 13 we are told the story of Jehoash, king of Israel. During battle, Jehoash sought the prophet Elisha's help. Elisha responded with a directive from God as to how to completely win a battle. Jehoash responded to that directive halfheartedly. As a result, he did not win the battle. The lesson from this brief passage of Scripture is clear. In order to receive the full benefits of God's plan for our lives, we must *fully* receive and obey His commands. If your child is learning self-control, begin by encouraging her to keep

TRYING TO DEVELOP SELF-CONTROL WITHOUT GOD'S HELP REQUIRES SELF-EFFORT AND OFTEN ENDS IN DEFEAT.

God's commands. Then allow His spirit to work a deep work in her day by day. The result will be one of the fruits of the Spirit listed in Galatians 5. This process is usually part of a child's development over time. Children are impulsive by nature and don't like to wait. They grow into maturity as they develop physically, emotionally, and spiritually. As they see their parents exhibiting the fruit of self-control, they will be encouraged by what God can do in them as they grow.

Empathy Is a Learned Trait

Some years ago, my sweet little girl asked a question that took me by surprise, not because she asked it but because of what she had noticed at such a young age. "Mom," she said, "No one wants to play with 'Sandy' because she is fat. That isn't right, is it? I felt bad for her."

"So what did you do?" I inquired, still shocked that she had made this observation at the ripe old age of five. "I told those kids my mom works with fat people and they better start being nice! Then I played with her."

It was a proud moment for her therapist mom. Yes, as an eating disorder therapist, I do work with overweight people. Consequently, I often talk with my family about the discrimination experienced by those who are obese and overweight, including the name-calling and teasing overweight people almost always endure. I tried to help them understand how much name-calling and teasing can hurt. Sticks and stones do break bones, but words hurt even more, sometimes for a lifetime. It was my wish that they not be a part of hurting people this way.

If they saw an overweight child being teased, standing by passively and allowing it to happen wasn't acceptable. Instead, they've been taught to take the lead and try to stop the mean behavior. So when my young daughter acted on that lesson (the hope of every parent), it was a moment to remember. What I say as a parent matters, even when I think my advice goes in one ear and out the other.

(Cont'd)

Kindergartners are already aware of body types and making play decisions based on them. It's a thought that still bothers me today, and I'm glad it bothered my daughter too. I didn't know Sandy's parents, but I hoped they would help her deal with this teasing and love her no matter what she weighed. And as a parent, I talked to those school kids about Sandy's giving character and the ever-present smile on her face. The unspoken message I hoped to convey was that Sandy is more than her weight—a lesson that can't be learned too early.

Teasing

Kids are blunt. They say what they think. And they aren't always kind. Teasing is one of the cruelest acts children can do to one another. Teasing can be brutal like, "Hey fatso! Can you squeeze into your desk?" or more subtle like, "Do you think you should eat that pizza?" And when teasing comes from family members, it has a much more devastating effect. Kids can become depressed, hate their bodies, and plummet in their self-esteem.

The truth is that overweight kids are teased more often than kids who are of average weight. One of the most common methods of teasing happens when a child is intentionally left out of social activities. And of course there is name-calling and physical shoves and pushes. Teasing is harmful to children in that it can result in feelings of rejection, discrimination, experienced failure with peer relationships, and limited group and social interests. Because of this, parents should make every effort to confront teasing when it happens.

We know that some children learn to effectively handle teasing and avoid being repeatedly victimized. Other children don't do as well and find themselves the brunt of much teasing. According to researchers, we still don't know exactly why some kids manage teasing better than others. I suspect it has to do with the personality of certain kids, their sensitivity levels, and the way they think. Overweight kids tend to describe themselves as less self-confident than average-weight kids. They know their weight makes them vulnerable to teasing and rejection.

A No-Tolerance Approach

All parents need to talk to their kids about the hurt teasing causes. Minimizing the impact of teasing is a bad idea—what seems like a small thing to you could be a big thing to your child—so it should not be ignored. So many adults in therapy today can still recall the name-calling and moments of teasing from their childhood. Teasing leaves a lasting impression and makes it necessary to take a no-tolerance approach.

If you hear an overweight child being tormented, confront the teasing child and make him apologize to the child he teased. Tell the teaser to stop this rude and disrespectful behavior as nothing justifies being cruel to another person. Ask the teasing child if he has ever been teased, and then ask how it felt. Then ask why he would want to do that very thing that felt so awful to another person. Explain what empathy is and also teach the child that he should treat others as he wants to be treated.

If the teasing child blankly stares at you, just say, "You need to stop hurting (insert name here). It isn't nice." Then tell the child that you will be watching him to see if he continues to tease. If, at another time, you see that child behaving appropriately with overweight kids, approach him and praise him. Tell him you saw how kind and nice he was. Point out that this is the person God wants him to be.

Earlier I said you don't want to minimize teasing. You also want to be careful not to overreact to teasing. If your child is teased, address it. Confront the teaser if necessary and deal with it, but don't make it bigger than it is for the moment. In other words, don't react out of your history of hurt. Instead, you want to convey to your child that the two of you will handle this and work on improving the situation. Be positive and give hope.

Jesus was teased and rejected for our sakes. I like to remind children that He knows what it feels like and can understand the pain. He died to carry that pain for us. We can pray and lay the hurt at His feet, forgiving those who have hurt us and allowing God to heal us. We can also find friends who are more sensitive and thoughtful of others. Encourage your child to find friends who are nice to be around and who don't tease. There are usually a few children known for their empathy and kindness of heart. Talk to your child about who those kids might be and invite them over to play.

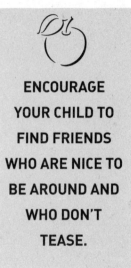

ENCOURAGE YOUR CHILD TO FIND FRIENDS WHO ARE NICE TO BE AROUND AND WHO DON'T TEASE.

When it comes to teasing, we parents are once again the role models. How we handle teasing will be noticed and modeled, so it's time for some self reflection. Ask yourself if you model being a victim. Do you carry grudges and talk about them in front of your children? Are you quick to blame others and feel defeated by the power of their words? Has the wounding in your own life remained unresolved, and is easily triggered by a negative remark? Do you feel as if you are in the victim position because of your weight, or for some other reason? If you do, take your areas of hurt and pain to God. Choose to forgive those who hurt you and ask God to heal those places inside.

Finally, be honest. Do you tease others? Do you make negative comments about other people's bodies and judge them? If you do, analyze why that is. Perhaps you are using teasing as a method to tell someone you have concerns about their weight, or any other characteristic. But teasing is not a "soft" way to peddle an opinion; direct conversation is much better.

To help your child, be open about the effects of teasing. When your child seems down, ask what is bothering him or her. Children won't automatically come to their parents when they have been hurt by teasing, and parents won't always notice like they would if there had been a physical battle. Follow these steps:

1. Gather as much information as you can about the specifics—who is doing what to whom? Is there a pattern, a specific time this happens, or something that usually prompts the teasing? How does your child react? Listen to your child's explanation.

2. Teach your child strategies to use (several are listed below) in order to empower her to act and not be a victim. Practice the strategies by using role-play.

3. Provide love and encouragement along the way, acknowledging that words can hurt if we let them. What's more, people can be mean and we can't always stop them—but we can pray for them and try to be like Christ in the way we respond. In the end, we are responsible for how we act, not for the actions of others.

4. Encourage your child to forgive those who have hurt her. Pray with her and tell her to verbalize who and why she needs to forgive. The feelings associated with forgiveness sometimes take time to catch up with the willful decision to do it. For example, she can say, "God, I am angry, but I choose to forgive Mary for saying those mean words to me." The important thing is not to let negative emotions like anger take hold and create bitterness.

5. Discuss teasing with teachers or other involved adults. It's important for children to know that when they've tried what they know to do and it has failed, a caring adult will step in and take charge.

Teasing in the Home

Jennifer sipped her cup of tea while the tears rolled down her face. She was visibly upset about her ex-husband's backhanded comment spoken to their eight-year-old daughter Amy earlier that day. Amy had picked out a special outfit to wear to a friend's birthday party. When she came out of her bedroom all dressed up, her dad glanced at her briefly from behind his newspaper and remarked, "That top is too tight and makes you look fat. Go change." Without a thought as to what this did to Amy's fragile esteem, he went back to reading the paper.

A Happy Ending

Tyler sat alone in his usual place on the playground. *If only recess would hurry up and be over,* he thought to himself. Fifth grade recess was a far cry from his first two years in elementary school. That was before his sister, Ann, became sick. Ann had been diagnosed with cancer and then died last year.

During the time of her illness, Tyler hurt in ways he had never hurt before. During mealtimes at home, no one talked when his sister was sick. The silence at the table was chilling. When Ann died, no one seemed to care about eating anymore. The dinner table became even more silent with the empty chair left where Ann used to sit.

All Tyler could say about his family life was that it felt lonely. His mom and dad were constantly sad, and he didn't know how to make them smile again. He had turned to food to help him get through his day when his sister was first diagnosed. As a result, Tyler gained a lot of weight, and now that his sister has passed away, he is still eating. But now the kids don't play with him at recess. He has tried to join in when there was an organized game of kickball, but the last comment he heard was enough to sideline him for good. "Hey, the fat kid needs to play! Don't get kicked by him or you'll be out like a light!"

Tyler felt the tears begin to well up in his eyes. He wouldn't cry in front of the other boys. He walked behind the school and cried alone. Humiliated, hurting, and alone, he made his way to his lunchbox and reached for the goodies he had bought with extra money. He missed his sister and he missed his parents, who seemed pretty oblivious to him, and life seemed pretty hopeless right now.

When the guidance counselor noticed Tyler sitting alone at recess for days and then weeks, she decided to call Tyler's mom. Were they aware of how sad Tyler appeared and how much weight he had gained since second grade? Mom admitted she had noticed the weight gain, but she didn't know what to do. She was struggling to help Tyler with

(Cont'd)

his grief because hers was so overwhelming. "Perhaps your family could come in and we could talk about all of this together?" the counselor suggested.

A bit relieved, Mom consented and the family worked on the grief related to Ann's death. It was the first time the family had talked about Ann together since she died. Then the counselor worked with the teachers to take a no-tolerance approach to verbal teasing. The counselor assigned an aid to listen for teasing on the playground. When teasing was heard, those kids responsible were brought to the counselor and made to apologize to the unfortunate person being teased. The teaser would have to sit out for recess if teasing remarks were made again. Then the counselor arranged for a "buddy" to be assigned to Tyler. The buddy would invite Tyler to play and spend time re-engaging him in recess again.

Tyler's parents worked hard at reconnecting with their son emotionally. They made mealtimes a time of nurturing and care once again. Now that the family could grieve together, they talked about their loss but also attended to the son who was living. Mom cooked healthy meals and soon Tyler's weight caught up to his height. The family had successfully regrouped over a painful loss, and Tyler's need to eat in order to fill the emptiness was no longer an issue. Unfortunately, not every story has a happy ending like Tyler's. Sadly, some of those kids may even try suicide.[1] In addition, kids who are overweight usually have fewer friends and tend to withdraw and isolate themselves from others.

Amy's eyes began to tear up and she ran back to her room. When she came home after her weekend of visitation, she relayed to her mom what Dad had said. She was crying. Jennifer was angry. *Yes, Amy was overweight, but did he have to be so insensitive?* All the unresolved feelings from the divorce began to well up in Jennifer. It was one thing for him to be a jerk to her, but for him to behave that way to their daughter was more than she could bear!

Jennifer isn't powerless over her ex-husband's insensitivity. She can confront him, explain the ill effects of his remarks, and ask him to stop creating esteem problems for their daughter. If he refuses, Jennifer can explain to Amy that her dad loves her but needs to work on controlling his mouth. When he says mean things, she will need to forgive him and pray that he will allow God to change his heart.

Jennifer can help her child feel loved and accepted no matter what is said. She will need to teach her daughter to appeal to a higher authority when it comes to image and acceptance. The words of a father are powerful in a child's life, but Amy's esteem will ultimately need to be based on how God thinks of her. Scriptures concerning her worth, unconditional love, and esteem will need to be read and prayed regularly. Hopefully, there will be other important men in Amy's life who will reinforce the message that Amy is more than her weight.

Is it unfair that Jennifer's ex-husband is an insensitive dad? Yes. But since that isn't something Jennifer and Amy have control over, they have to accept it and move on. Jennifer and her daughter have choices to make about how they respond to those unfair circumstances and people. They can give such people undue power in their lives or take action where and when they can. Even though Jennifer's ex-husband is a powerful influence over their daughter, Jennifer is also a powerful voice in Amy's life. With God's help, the study of scriptures on esteem, healing prayer, and other positive male influences, Jennifer's daughter can learn to feel good about herself regardless of her father's inane comments. This will be a process accomplished over time with God's help.

When teasing comes from within the family, confront the behavior. Tell that family member this is not a nice way to act, that it does not imitate Christ nor reflect the values of your family. Ask that person to stop and apologize to the teased child. Then talk to the teaser about why he would do such a thing. Get to the heart of the issue and try to resolve it. For example, if a sibling is jealous, find out why and help her resolve those feelings. If an ex-spouse wants to get back at his wife by hurting their child, he needs counseling help.

If the teaser is a spouse, point out the consequences of the continued behavior to the child. Remind the spouse that he is setting the child up for problems now and in the future. Teasing hurts—whether intended or unintended. Words are powerful! Proverbs 18:21 clearly instructs us that the tongue has the power of life or death in it. Words can hurt and can't be retracted. In fact, the Bible tells us we will be judged for every word we speak. A teasing spouse should ask himself, "Are my words building up my child or tearing her down?" If the answer is the latter, that spouse has a problem that needs intervention. Anyone who would willfully hurt their child after being confronted about it needs to be held accountable and directed to counseling.

The first step in correcting a hurtful tongue is to ask for forgiveness. Then a person must be willing to change. True change is a matter of the heart. It comes in response to God as one confesses sin and asks the Holy Spirit to empower a change in speech. Self-control is a fruit of the Spirit and results as we abide in Christ.

If you are dealing with a family member who refuses to change and has no interest in spiritual matters, you will need to stay on top of what is being said and correct those statements with your child. Tell her that what was said is not true and that you are sorry that person was hurtful. Ask if she is willing to forgive what was said and then pray

What to Do

Ask if your child is being teased. Some kids won't bring up the subject unless you ask. If teasing is happening, you will want to talk through ways to handle it, pray with your child, and remind her that what other children say about her is not always true. Instill the truth that there are no physical qualifiers for being accepted by God.

that the negative words will bear no fruit in your child's life. Pray the healing words of Scripture God brings to you with and over your child, always reminding her of her true identity.

Teasing Outside the Home

Unfortunately, there are children in our culture who lack empathy and do not listen to their moral conscience. Whether they have had no religious training or haven't been taught to respect others, it is a sad reality that children can be very unkind. Many come from homes in which they are teased and bullied and learn to do the same behavior to other children. Not all teasing can be stopped. As a result, you will need to equip your child with other strategies to handle teasing when it happens. Here are a number of options. Have your child consider these ten alternatives:

1. Encourage your child not to respond to teasing with violence. He can defend himself if a child becomes physical, but encourage him to respond with words first in order to resolve conflicts. You may have to role-play situations and practice specifically what your child can say. Have your child practice how she would answer someone who teased her.

   Give her a suggestion like, "Look, you need to stop. What you are doing is mean and wrong." Have your child wait a minute and see what happens. If the other child continues to tease, have your child say, "If you don't stop, I'm getting an adult. It's up to you." If the other child doesn't stop, then it's time to find an adult and ask the adult to intervene.

2. Consider the possibility that your child may be inciting teasing without knowing it. Some overweight kids can say provocative things to get attention. Others may be wearing clothing that doesn't fit because they have outgrown it. It's always a good idea to ask your child if she is being teased for reasons other than her weight. This doesn't in any way excuse teasing, but it may help her see she can bring undue negative attention to herself by acting in inappropriate

ways. For example, if your daughter constantly complains about other children, other children may pick on her. Her weight may have little to do with the teasing, yet other kids will make the weight the target of their teasing. In those cases, you have to help your child connect her actions to the behavior of others.

3. Help your child understand that while we can't control what others say and do, we can control how we react. Teach him to take the high road and imitate Christ in all he does. This is not easy for a child. Pray for the bullies and those who tease. Then discuss how important it is to not stoop to their unkind behavior or imitate them.

4. Contact the parent of the teaser and try to discuss ways to help both children. You can't do this if you feel angry or hostile, because the other parent will become defensive. So wait until you feel in control of your feelings. Simply state the behavior and then ask if the parent has any idea what might be going on and why this is happening. Tell the parent you would like to find a way to work out the problem so both kids will get along and be respectful to each other.

   You won't always get cooperation with this strategy. Sometimes kids tease other kids because they are being teased at home. And of course, there is always the parent who thinks her child is an angel despite the evidence.

5. Coach your child to use humor to take the punch out of teasing. Many kids will stop teasing someone once they see they don't get the reaction they wanted from the person being teased. Humor can deflect the tension and may work if your child can come up with a funny comeback.

6. A child can counter teasing by using his self-talk to say, "I don't need to listen to this; what is being said isn't true." He can then walk away if necessary.

7. Ignore the teasing. Most times, this strategy will work because the other child doesn't get a reaction. Encourage your child to try to

ignore the teasing and see what happens. Yet even if ignoring works to stop the teasing, ask your child how she feels about what was said. You may still need to help her not accept those words as truth in terms of what was said.

8. A strategy that works for some children is to visualize the hurtful words bouncing off of them like a shield. Spiritually, you can teach a child about using the shield of faith in a visual way. When he is being verbally attacked, he can visualize his shield of faith going up and the words falling away.

9. Respond with the following: "So?" It communicates an indifference to the words spoken, and it works because the teaser doesn't get the reaction he is hoping to get.

10. Ask for help. When a child is feeling overwhelmed or hurt by teasing, it's best to ask for help so that adults can become involved. This is not a sign of weakness or "ratting" another child out. Rude behavior should be stopped because of the harm it causes to another. Adults should intervene and provide consequences for someone who continues to tease.

Teasing doesn't always stop, even with intervention, because we can't force other people to be sensitive or have empathy. But there is much you can do to prepare your child so that she can respond appropriately and not be defined by the teasing. Problem-solving and being assertive can go a long way to empower a child. Equally helpful is the reality that children tend to worry less when they know parents are aware of a problem. As parents we have the opportunity to provide our children with a framework to think about teasing and how to respond to others, which is effectively training our children for life.

One of the most difficult lessons to be learned is to love our enemies, bless those who curse us, do good to those who hate us, and pray for those who spitefully use and persecute us (Matthew 5:44). Jesus' teaching in this area is radical to our flesh nature and to the larger culture's response, and almost impossible to do without His Spirit

> AS PARENTS, WE HAVE AN OPPOR-TUNITY TO TRAIN AND EQUIP OUR CHILDREN EARLY ON WITH GODLY PRINCIPLES THAT WILL BRING HEALING TO THEIR SOULS.

abiding in us. Yet there is tremendous power and peace in following Christ's words and putting His teachings into practice. As parents, we have an opportunity to train and equip our children early on with godly principles that will bring healing to their souls. Help your child confess the hurt, forgive the person who hurt him, and pray for the love of God to be revealed to that person.

Dealing with Bullies

Overweight kids have a good chance of encountering a bully, especially at school.

The National School Safety Center calls "bullying" the most enduring and under-rated problem in American schools. Kids identified as bullies by age eight are three times as likely as other youths to break the law by age thirty.[2] Obviously, early intervention is the key.

Here's a typical encounter. Your fifth-grade son is playing soccer on the playground at recess. A sixth grade bully comes over and takes his ball, throws it at him, and laughs as he walks away. What should your son do?

A. Throw the ball back at him.

B. Walk away and say nothing.

C. Report the boy to school authorities.

D. Go after the kid and try to talk to him.

Do you want to phone a friend before your final answer? Dads tend to choose answer *A* because they want their son to fight back and show

REPORTING A BULLY SHOULD BE VIEWED MORE AS AN ACT OF LOVE THAN ANYTHING ELSE—ONCE A BULLY IS IDENTIFIED, HE CAN GET HELP.

the bully he'll have someone to contend with if he continues the mean behavior. Moms like *D* because women tend to think we can solve these things by talking them out. Answer *B* is good if you can get your son to do it; however, walking away does nothing to correct the bully's behavior. So that leaves us with answer *C*.

Reporting a bully is sometimes unpopular because kids fear revenge and being labeled a tattletale, but bullies need to be reported. School authorities should become involved, because this sort of behavior leaves a potential window for violence, and kids need the protection and authority of school officials. Reporting a bully should be viewed more as an act of love than anything else— once a bully is identified, he can get help.

What you don't want is for your child to harbor anger and look for ways to take revenge or get even. These options may be encouraged by people who lack faith as they are not Christlike responses. Ask your child to write down bully situations on 3 x 5 cards; more than likely, he will come up with examples in no time. Then role-play the situations and practice different ways to handle a specific problem. Talk about why some solutions are good choices and others aren't so good. Role-playing gives children a plan of action so they can be more confident when the encounter occurs.

The Heart of the Matter

When children feel bad about their bodies and weight, it is because they believe things about themselves that may or may not be true. Behind every weight problem is a thought about that problem that may or may not be based in truth. For example, *I am teased because of my weight,* is a true thought that causes a child to feel anger, sadness, or hurt. If your child shares such thoughts and feelings, he can ask Jesus to carry that pain. Assure him that Jesus died on the cross and takes all our hurts and pains onto Himself.

Lead your child in a simple prayer like, "Jesus, please take my hurt. I don't want it and You can take it." Then ask the child if there is anything else he may want to do. Often children will tell you they need to forgive the person who hurt them. If he doesn't suggest this, take the initiative and ask directly, "Do you need to forgive (insert name) for hurting you?" Then lead your child in a prayer of forgiveness and ask for that person to be more loving.

Once your child has expressed the hurt, given it to God, and prayed to forgive the person who hurt him, reassure your child that you love him. Tell him we can't always stop people from doing or saying negative things, but we can choose not to let them have power over us by confronting the bad feelings and letting go of them and forgiving the people who hurt us. Also reassure him that you will do what you can to help stop teasing behavior.

If the emotional pain your child feels is related to a lie he believes about himself, provide examples of the truth found in God's Word and those things that you know to be true of your son. Tell him, "Here is what God says about you (list four or five specifics from Scripture)." Then tell him what you know to be true. List another four or five examples and then broaden the list to include statements from others who know your child well. In other words, provide evidence that will counter the lie.

For example, if a classmate called your child a "Fat Pig" and she comes home crying, ask your daughter how she is feeling. She will probably say she is hurting, sad, or angry. Then ask why she feels that way. If she tells you what happened, ask how true she thinks those hurtful words are. And if she says the words are very true or that she agrees with those words or thinks they might be true, say, "Honey, here's what God says about you (use your list). Here's what I say about you (use your list), and here's what (name a number of people who know your child) say about you. Who are you going to believe? The words of another child who is being mean or the words of those who love and know you?"

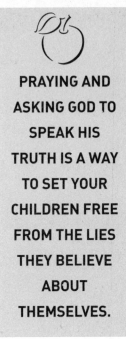

PRAYING AND ASKING GOD TO SPEAK HIS TRUTH IS A WAY TO SET YOUR CHILDREN FREE FROM THE LIES THEY BELIEVE ABOUT THEMSELVES.

Praying and asking God to speak His truth is a way to set your children free from the lies they believe about themselves. The earlier you can tackle these lies that tend to become implanted, the better. You can help your child gain a truthful perspective about who she is in Christ Jesus and remind her how others see her as well. No matter how many times we tell our children how much they are loved and accepted by God, they need reassurance when someone questions their worth or value.

This is my prayer for you and your children:

God, help each person who reads this to be encouraged by the hope that is in You. There is no problem too difficult for You to solve. As we put our trust in You, You will give each of us the wisdom and discernment we need to provide positive, practical, and spiritual help to our children. Speak your truth to those places in our minds that have been filled with lies. Don't allow teasing and hurt to create a stronghold of anger or depression. Help each child to know the truth and be set free by it. Thank You for being true to Your promises and faithful in our lives. Amen.

POINTS TO PONDER

1. Encourage a biblical approach to developing self-control.

2. Teasing is a cruel reality of life, and we need to be ready for it and also recognize how powerful it is.

3. Equip your child with options to handle teasing and practice them with role-play.

4. Help renew the mind of a child who has been teased or rejected. Allow God's truth to penetrate her soul.

10

Schools Do Play a Role

The Rogers family lives a busy life. Every morning all three children get ready for school while Mom and Dad get ready for work. The bus comes early and the entire family is out of the house by 7:45 a.m. As busy as life is right now, there is no time to eat breakfast or pack lunches, and so all three boys eat both of those meals at school. School meals are inexpensive and convenient, which is what the parents appreciate. The boys like the food and are eager to purchase doughnuts for fifty cents each at breakfast, and pizza or hot dogs for seventy-five cents at lunch.

The problem is that one of the boys, Jack, is gaining weight. Even though Mrs. Rogers only works part-time and is home in plenty of time to cook a nutritious dinner, breakfasts and lunches are eaten at school, away from her watchful eye. Because the boys are utilizing the federally regulated school lunch and breakfast program, Mrs. Rogers doesn't give much thought to the reality that her son's diet is in fact very unhealthy. When she does investigate into the school's programs and the options her kids have for meals, she is aghast at what the boys are eating.

Jack is so hungry some mornings that he buys three to four doughnuts. During lunchtime, he often eats a piece of pizza and a hot dog and washes it down with a large soda purchased from the vending machine in the hallway. Jack's

(Cont'd)

> *older brother loaned him money for the vending machines in*
> *exchange for doing some of his chores—a deal unknown to*
> *the parents. In addition, other kids who purchase snacks*
> *from the vending machines frequently share their goodies*
> *with Jack. By the time Jack returned home from school, he*
> *had consumed a high number of calories with little nutri-*
> *tional value. And he was still hungry and ready for a big*
> *dinner! Mrs. Rogers now knew exactly why Jack was*
> *gaining weight.*

Before she investigated Jack's school eating habits, Mrs. Rogers had no idea that the school had installed vending machines and that school breakfasts included doughnuts. She regularly reviewed the weekly school menu online but learned much later that à la carte food was also available for purchase. Her boys could skip the meal tray of eggs and toast and buy doughnuts instead. The lunches offered included the standard school tray described in the school menu, but again, high-fat fast food was also provided by a local fast-food chain. Jack admitted that he often traded his lunch tray for hot dogs and pizza.

Meet Kelly, a second grader who lives with her grandparents. Kelly is an excellent student and gets straight *A's* on her report card. Last semester Kelly was rewarded for her excellent grades through a school incentive program. A local baker offered a free doughnut for every *A* on Kelly's report card. When Kelly rushed home with news about this incentive program, her grandparents became upset with the school. Kelly, along with several of her classmates, is overweight and doesn't need doughnuts as a reward for her good grades. Kelly's grandparents are working hard to provide Kelly with rewards that do not include food. Given the fact that so many kids are overweight in Kelly's school, it is puzzling that another incentive program wasn't implemented. Doesn't the school see that this program will undercut the grandparents' and other parents' efforts and likely contribute to Kelly's and other children's weight gain?

The Truth

As you can see from the above two stories, even schools aren't free from the tentacles of marketers and advertisers. When schools offer fast food and other tempting goodies, as well as sugary sodas out of vending machines, such foods take the place of nutritious meals needed for children to grow up healthy. Schools are contributing to the rising tide of overweight kids.

Once children reach school age, they spend a good part of their day at school. In terms of eating, children consume about one-third of their total daily calories at school. Since many kids buy both breakfast and lunch at school, they can easily be eating high-calorie, high-fat dense meals with little or no nutritional value. Even though the U.S. Department of Agriculture's National School Lunch/Breakfast program must follow federal nutrition guidelines, kids can purchase "competitive" foods which are not regulated. These foods are often offered as à la carte items, or they are found in school vending machines.

You may be wondering why junk and fast foods are even allowed in the schools. Sadly, it boils down to money! With more budget cuts, schools have turned to private companies to fund a number of budget line items. This means schools are in the business of selling fast foods and vending products in order to make money to underwrite their budgets. According to the CDC, 73.9 percent of middle schools have either vending machines or snack bars where high-calorie foods and soft drinks are sold. The number increases to a whopping 98.2 percent when kids reach high school.

Advertisements for candy, soft drinks, and fast foods are allowed in more than 20 percent of schools.[1] Schools work deals with soft drink companies in order to obtain a percentage of the sales.[2] Believe it or not, Coca-Cola Enterprises Inc. is a "proud" sponsor of the National PTAs Parent Involvement School Certification program![3] How incredible is that? The national PTA, an organization whose mission is supposed to be to support and speak out for children and their welfare, is sponsored by Coca-Cola! The justification is that schools need this additional revenue in order to buy needed equipment and other products cut from school budgets. It's an old and tired argument: the means justify the end—even at the expense of our children's health.

Having soft drinks available at schools only contributes to consumption. The data shows that between 56 and 85 percent of children drink sodas every day![4] Filled with sugar, caffeine, and empty calories, such drinks do not help our children deal with weight problems or the growing rate of type 2 diabetes. It's hard to rationalize the fact that schools will fund programs through the use of unhealthy products for kids. The real question is, what's more important—the health of our children or the number of computers in a classroom? The answer is obvious.

When faced with the decision to either buy pizza and Coke and a Snickers Bar or the healthy milk, fish, and vegetables on the school tray, what would you choose if you were an eleven-year-old? Even when parents make a point of teaching their children not to purchase unhealthy items at school, kids are still bombarded with ads, unhealthy fast food available right in the cafeteria, and conveniently placed vending machines in the halls. And while parents *can* teach their kids to make healthy choices, it isn't easy when all the other kids are munching on fries. When children are young, it's easier to help them restrain their eating because parents are the money source. However, as they get older, it's more difficult because children have their own money earned from chores and special occasions and can purchase items on their own. Having the items so readily available at school means parents can quite easily be left out of the loop.

When marketers do their job right, kids see these unhealthy products and want to buy them. The problem is that young children don't have the cognitive capacity to understand persuasive intent by advertisers. They look at an ad or a commercial, see the happy, popular, or sexy person recommending the product, and are enticed by the clever animation or marketing angle to believe they need that product or should eat it. Junk food is an easy sell because it's relatively cheap, appealing to the taste, and leaves no evidence (other than fat cells) for parents to find and ask about.

Another problem is that kids are developmentally impulsive and focused on the immediate. They don't think long term about their health. That's the job of grown-ups! We certainly aren't helping them by allowing advertisers and marketers to invade our schools with unhealthy products.

One of the practical steps you can take is to pack your child's lunch every day and reinforce his need to eat what is sent to school. This way, you have some control over what he eats at lunch. You may have to wake up earlier and plan ahead in order to pack lunches. Have your children help you decide what they would like in their lunches the night before and get the lunch boxes out and ready to go. Many schools have microwave ovens so you can even send portions of leftover meals or soup in thermos containers. Encourage your children not to trade their lunches— they need to eat what Mom and Dad have packed for them.

ONE OF THE PRACTICAL STEPS YOU CAN TAKE IS TO PACK YOUR CHILD'S LUNCH EVERY DAY AND REINFORCE HIS NEED TO EAT WHAT IS SENT TO SCHOOL.

What Parents Can Do

Currently, there are a number of bills on the table to get unhealthy products out of the schools. There are also activist groups trying to make changes. It is the responsibility of every parent to be informed as to what their children have access to in the schools. Yes, there are federal programs which do regulate the nutritional lunches being served, but there are other foods that have no need to be regulated being served in the same room! If your school is placing vending machines, selling candy, and offering fast-food alternatives for lunches, meet with administrators and tell them your feelings about this. You have a tax-paying right to challenge their decisions. You could be instrumental in removing these machines from your child's school!

Got Lunch?

Lunch box suggestions for both kids and adults include fresh fruits, crunchy vegetables, slices of lean meat, hard-boiled eggs, peanut butter (put it on the veggies), cheese slices, yogurt, crackers, and flat bread, pita, or other whole-grain breads or rolls. To keep lunches from getting boring, use a variety of foods and mix them up daily. Insulated containers are great for soups or healthy leftovers. Also include a water bottle so your kids aren't tempted to drink soda.

Los Angeles parent Arely Herrera joined a grassroots group of parents, teachers, administrators, and students who were concerned about the food being offered in their school. This group teamed up with Occidental College's Center for Food and Justice, a group that worked to provide nutritious food programs for schools. Together they formed the Healthy School Food Coalition (HSFC). For three years the coalition campaigned to get salad bars and other healthier snacks into schools. They surveyed parents, spoke at school board meetings, presented petitions, sampled cafeteria food, and presented alternatives to the current foods offered. They eventually won their battle. Ms. Herrera credits the work of prepared and aggressive parents who cared about the growing obesity problem in the schools.[5]

Another parent, Turusew Gedebu-Wilson, dietitian and mom of a child in a California school, heard that the school's breakfast and lunch programs were not nutritionally great. She began to check into the situation and offered to help improve the menus. Writing for the school newsletter and getting parents involved resulted in changes and improvements in both meals the schools served.[6] One parent can make a difference.

Parents do have a voice that can be used effectively to advocate change. Start by building relationships with local school personnel and be involved in your child's school. You will have a better chance of being heard and having school personnel cooperate with you. Let school personnel know that you would like to work with them to make changes. You have the best interest of your child in mind. Form a working partnership and encourage other parents to be involved as well.

What Schools Can Do—and Are Doing

All across our nation, over eight million students in 12,000 schools are exposed to two minutes of advertisements imbedded in a twelve-minute news segment from an in-school television network called Channel One. Primemedia, an independent news media outlet, delivers this program to our kids through schools. Here's how it works: If a school signs up for Channel One, they receive $50,000 worth of telecommunications equipment that becomes the school's property after six years of using the service. The equipment includes a fixed KU band satellite dish, nineteen-inch color televisions for every classroom, VCRs and internal wiring, and complete maintenance by Channel One.[7]

The twelve-minute daily news program offers educational, training, and student programming. The two minutes of daily commercials finance the program. However, the controversy over this "service" is so strong that some schools have made the decision to shut down the program. The issue is the invasion of commercialism into the schools and the content of ads and media advertised. In terms of kids and weight, much of the controversy centers on the fact that sodas and junk food are advertised, promoting unhealthy food choices and lifestyle habits. Pediatrician Dr. Carden Johnston criticized Channel One's ads because they promote soft drinks and candy and conflict with the foods regulated by the National School Lunch Program.[8] And with the epidemic of obesity we have on our hands, food advertisements on school time isn't a justifiable option.

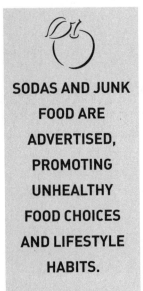

SODAS AND JUNK FOOD ARE ADVERTISED, PROMOTING UNHEALTHY FOOD CHOICES AND LIFESTYLE HABITS.

The bigger question is: "what about the health and welfare of our children?" Unfortunately, kids are big business. Channel One has been so successful that other companies are following their lead. ZapMe! is one of those companies. This corporation offers to loan fifteen computers and accessories free of charge to any school. They provide the software, Netspace, that allows students to visit up to 10,000 Internet websites they have approved. Netspace also allows students to have personal email at school. That's right, personal email that can be sent and received!

In order to receive the equipment, the school must agree to have students utilize the computers for at least four hours of every day. During that time, ZapMe! Advertisements are constantly running on a part of the computer screen. Students can click on an ad anytime and enlarge it.[9] The ads are aimed at altering the buying habits and lifestyle choices of young people. These commercials encourage materialism, already a problem among our children, and also market unhealthy products that contribute to obesity, poor nutrition, and eating disorders.

Stop the Madness

You don't have to be an activist to see the relationship between the welfare of kids and the commercialism aimed their direction. Advertisers are purposely targeting younger and younger kids knowing that they influence family spending, are future consumers, and often have their own money to spend. Marketers know kids are easily influenced when it comes to consumerism. Recent studies show that by the time American kids are three years old, they can recognize an average of one hundred brand logos.[10]

This madness must stop. It's working against what we know is best for kids. It's time to care more about our nation's children than the profit earned by exploiting them. Your part is to stay on top of what is being offered in your schools. When you become aware of a problem, write letters, talk to administrators, protest advertising to children in school—it's exploitative of your children, not to mention the fact that it takes away from school learning time and trains them to value material things.

Advertising and Kids

It is the goal of most kid marketers to become a part of the fabric of children's lives. If they can "surround" market a child, meaning capture a child's attention at every possible moment, then they can sell more products. Sadly, psychologists are often hired to help these advertisers find effective ways to persuade our children to buy their unhealthy products. The result is a growing tension between Mom and Dad and the advertisers peddling those products most parents oppose.

When your child brings home the doughnut coupon for good grades, trade it for a coupon that gives him exclusive time with Mom and Dad while doing some special activity. If your child begs for products offered in schools, say no and remain firm, no matter how much he begs or whines. Let him be upset while you explain the value of good health and taking care of your body. Teach him that there are many choices to make in life, and not all of the options are equally good. Pepsi and chips don't help children grow healthy and strong. Kids can cry and complain all they want, but parents have their welfare in mind.

Work with your school to implement the Childhood Obesity Prevention Agenda that has been endorsed by many leading obesity researchers and public health groups. This campaign was initiated in 2003 by Commercial Alert, a non-profit organization dedicated to banning the marketing, distribution, and sale of junk food in schools, and improving the quality of food provided to schoolchildren. Commercial Alert believes schools should support parents who are trying to instill good eating habits in their children, and corporations should not intrude on that territory. Furthermore, schools should promote healthy eating habits and exercise rather than junk food and other poor nutritional foods marketed by corporations.

Encourage your congressman or congresswoman to support the Parent's Bill of Rights (see below) which bans marketing to kids under twelve years of age, mandates disclosure of product placement, and revokes the tax subsidy that corporations receive for marketing to children.

Bring Back PE and Recess

Unfortunately, in many communities, non-academic programs like health education, physical education and even recess suffer or are elimi-

What Happened to Nutrition Class?

Healthy nutrition was once taught in home economics or health class. This is no longer the case in many schools. Efforts to keep junk food marketers out of the schools were lost in 1989 when Channel One launched its advertisements. Now schools trade Coke for cash and have become one of our biggest pushers of sodas. Perhaps it's time to educate our students and bring back classes that teach healthy nutrition.

The Parent's Bill of Rights[12]

WHEREAS, the nurturing of character and strong values in children is one of the most important functions of any society;

WHEREAS, the primary responsibility for the upbringing of children resides in their parents;

WHEREAS, an aggressive commercial culture has invaded the relationship between parents and children, and has impeded the ability of parents to guide the upbringing of their own children;

WHEREAS, corporate marketers have sought increasingly to bypass parents, and speak directly to children in order to tempt them with the most sophisticated tools that advertising executives, market researchers and psychologists can devise;

WHEREAS, these marketers tend to glorify materialism, addiction, hedonism, violence and anti-social behavior, all of which are abhorrent to most parents;

WHEREAS, parents find themselves locked in constant battle with this pervasive influence, and are hard pressed to keep the commercial culture and its degraded values out of their children's lives;

WHEREAS, the aim of this corporate marketing is to turn children into agents of corporations in the home, so that they will nag their parents for the things they see advertised, thus sowing strife, stress and misery in the family;

WHEREAS, the products advertised generally are ones parents themselves would not choose for their children: violent and sexually suggestive entertainment, video games, alcohol, tobacco, gambling and junk food;

WHEREAS, this aggressive commercial influence has contributed to an epidemic of marketing-related diseases in children, such as obesity, type 2 diabetes, alcoholism, anorexia and bulimia, while millions will eventually die from the marketing of tobacco;

WHEREAS, corporations have latched onto the schools and compulsory school laws as a way to bypass parents and market their products and values to a captive audience of impressionable and trusting children;

WHEREAS, these corporations ultimately are creatures of state law, and it is intolerable that they should use the rights and powers so granted for the purpose of undermining the authority of parents in these ways;

THEREFORE, BE IT RESOLVED, that the U.S. Congress and the fifty state legislatures should right the balance between parents and corporations and restore to parents some measure of control over the commercial influences on their children, by enacting this Parent's Bill of Rights . . .

nated altogether. These changes are significant for kids and their overall health. Less than 10 percent of schools now offer a daily PE program![12] That is a shocking statistic! Kids need to be *more* active. Dropping PE from their day means they are not getting exercise they desperately need.

In addition, many schools have shortened or eliminated recess time for elementary children. Again, this is not a good policy decision, as children need to have time to get up from their desks and move around. Sitting all day in a classroom is difficult for even the best-behaved children, not to mention encouraging our children to be sedentary. Recess provides a necessary release and should be included in the school day. For young children, there should be recesses in both mornings and afternoons.

Too Much Homework and Not Enough Play

Another way schools contribute to the growing problem of obesity is by assigning young children too much homework. After sitting all day in a classroom, often without PE or recess, children are then expected to go home and sit for another two to three hours to do homework. The homework overload has become so problematic in some schools that children literally move from the school building to their homework stations, and work late into the night.

If you feel your child has too much homework, consider these two options before approaching the teacher:

- Is your child taking too much on, whether because he was overly ambitious or because too much was expected of him by you, his parents? Parents should be sensitive to their children's schedules. If you are pushing your sixth grader to take French even though your child is struggling with it and frustrated with the language and falling behind, resulting in more homework and stress, perhaps the class should be dropped.

- Is your child utilizing all the work time that is offered at school? Is he studying during study hall, and is he trying to complete his homework when class time is given for that purpose? Don't be afraid to ask other parents if their children are feeling equally burdened with homework. Sometimes our children aren't working when they should be.

If you feel the problem is not one of the scenarios above, then it is time to speak with the teacher. Set up a conference, and if necessary, enlist the support of other parents. If changes don't result, meet with principles or administrators. When you have exhausted these resources, it is time to go to the school board.

Granted, all of this takes time and energy, but it is important for children to have balance. Kids need time to rest, play, and engage in other non-school activities such as music, dance, sports, reading for fun, and doing activities with their families. I've heard many children say they can't play a sport in school because there just isn't time to do all the homework required and be a good student while also playing a sport.

Sound Familiar?

"Amber" is a bright sixth grader who works at a good speed and stays on task. She turns in all assignments on time and, when possible, works ahead on projects so that she can finish tasks in an orderly fashion. She is highly organized and responsible.

Recently, her mom and dad watched her diligently attack an English assignment. It took everything in her to finish—over two hours' worth of time! Then she had to complete a French paper and study for a science test. At 10:15 p.m., she finally finished and was exhausted. Her bedtime is regularly 9:00 p.m. on school nights. The homework load was just too much, with the consequence being she had to sit in a chair all day and all evening and only focus on schoolwork. Furthermore, she told her parents that she is beginning to not like school, a problem they have never had with this child. If the homework load doesn't change, she'll be burned out by seventh grade!

This shouldn't be the case. For kids who are overweight, excessive homework is just one more sedentary activity contributing to the problem.

The Bottom Line

The bottom line is that schools need to start using common sense. At a time when obesity rates are climbing, a priority should be put on physical education, recess, and other activities that promote balance and a healthy lifestyle. More budget money and extra computers aren't worth having kids blatantly exploited by big corporations. Helping children grow up healthy is the responsibility of not only the parents but also the community at large. The messages being sent to our children through the school do not represent this reality.

Parents have to be aware of the unhealthy school influences that contribute to obesity and do everything possible to eliminate those influences. In practical terms, this means talking to kids about advertising and its purposes. As a family, discuss unhealthy products and what they do to the body. Teach your children to make wise choices, even when you aren't there. Pack lunches and snacks and monitor how much money your kids have in order to help them resist buying meals and snacks from vending machines.

POINTS TO PONDER

1. Walk the halls of your child's school. Look for soda and vending machines. If they exist, become a parent advocate and write to administrators to remove them. Speak up in your PTA and at school board meetings. Set rules about these machines with your children.

2. Check the nutritional value of the school lunch program. Pack your child a lunch if you are concerned. Work with the school to bring in more healthy foods.

3. Advocate for physical education, recess, and reasonable amounts of homework.

11

Media's Part in the Equation

"Did you hear Mary Kate went to a hospital because she wouldn't eat?"

"Yes, but my mom says it wasn't really a hospital like where we had our tonsils out, but a hospital where they help people eat because they are unhappy about a lot of things in their lives."

"How could Mary Kate be unhappy? Look at all the money she has. She's rich and famous and can have anything she wants. I would die for her wardrobe."

"My mom says that money doesn't always make people happy. I mean, look at all the movies, books, dolls, music, posters, and everything Mary Kate and Ashley have and she still had to go to that special kind of hospital."

"You know she does look pretty skinny on that poster in your room. I could never look like her. Sometimes that makes me sad."

"My mom says we shouldn't try to look like her. That we are just right the way we are."

"But she's so beautiful and has all that stuff."

"Yeah, but she's sick and needs help eating."

"Maybe we shouldn't try to be skinny like her. I don't want to go to a hospital and have people make me eat."

"What about Ashley? She's skinny too and she's not in a hospital."

(Cont'd)

> *"My mom said it's kind of complicated but that we shouldn't try to be like someone else. And we really shouldn't try to make ourselves skinny like those movie stars. I guess some famous people do bad things to their bodies to be skinny."*
>
> *"Like what?"*
>
> *"I don't know. I didn't ask."*
>
> *"Well, I might ask because I've been thinking I should go on a diet."*
>
> *"What? Why would you do that?"*
>
> *"To look like Mary Kate and Ashley. I think I look too fat."*
>
> *"But you're fine the way you are. Just because you aren't skinny like Mary Kate doesn't mean you're fat."*
>
> *"Well, maybe I won't try to be real skinny then. Maybe I'll just be normal me."*

The above conversation took place between two ten-year-old girls after they saw an article in the newspaper with Mary Kate Olsen's picture. For those of you who may not know who Mary Kate and Ashley are, they are the adorable twins made known to most of us from their early TV sitcom days with the show *Full House*. Since then, they have amassed a media empire worth about 300 million dollars. Together these famous twins own and manage several product lines. The newspaper heading read, "Mary Kate Olsen seeks treatment for an eating disorder."

Since the two ten-year-olds were fans of the Olsen twins (having seen every one of their movies), they were curious about the newspaper story.

Perhaps you've heard conversations like the one above with your own children. If so, listen carefully as conversations provide great clues as to how media influences the thinking of your children, especially when it comes to weight and body image.

Happily, one of these girls has been getting some great counsel from her mom about the media—and she is passing it on to her friend. Parents have great influence. Unfortunately, so does the media. Whether through glamorous images in magazines or time spent playing media, our kids' minds and bodies are impacted. However, parent influence matters more and can counter negative messages of media. When it comes to learning how to be responsible with media, parents are the primary teachers.

Weapons of Mass Seduction

Music and symbols. Fashion and materialism. American pop culture infiltrates the lives of young people through the mass media of television, Internet, music, movies, magazines, and more. MTV, an international television network, sells its explosive brand and lifestyle by promoting themes that influence an entire segment of our population. The Internet is no different in this regard—image obsession becomes idol worship on the worldwide converged network. Physical appearance, especially as modeled by media, is of paramount importance. Kids are often judged by their peers in terms of culturally defined standards of beauty and fashion that is actually set by the world's mass media.

Technology now influences our children in ways never seen before. If you think about all the screens kids sit in front of on a regular basis, it isn't hard to see why children aren't getting enough physical exercise. Television, computers, video games, PDAs, and electronic games all vie for our children's time and attention. Kids are avid consumers of media, to the tune of an average 40 hours a week.[1] Time once spent outside and running around the neighborhood or in imaginative play is now spent in front of media screens. Consequently, we need to pay attention to what messages are being sent and how they impact children.

I have a television, and my children do watch it. I'm not one of those parents who has thrown out the TV and banned all electronics. Media can be used to entertain and educate our children in ways that are absolutely delightful. Most parents recognize the usefulness of media in our children's lives as well as our own. However, media can become problematic when it is consumed in excess. Equally troubling is the reality that many children are unsupervised when it comes to discerning what is appropriate for their age group. Children should not be responsible for sifting the messages they are being fed—that is the responsibility of the parents. The quality and content of both television shows and Internet websites children frequent should be familiar territory for parents.

Though regulations are in place, that fact seems to have little effect in stopping the messages our kids pick up from TV. Sadly, many producers of television and other media do not seem to care about the health of our children. There is blatant disregard for the data that supports the harm they help perpetuate among children. As a parent, be vigilant and take an interest in the media your child sees in order to combat the lies being peddled to children.

The Thin Ideal

When it comes to our bodies, both children and adults get a mixed message from pop culture and advertisements. On the one hand, we are told that being thin and beautiful is the key to success. On the other, we are bombarded with messages to consume unhealthy, fattening foods and engage in unhealthy lifestyles that lead to a weight problem. The message is: be thin, but eat whatever and whenever you feel like it! How mixed up is that? It's all enough to make any sane person a little crazy and confused!

Since WWII, our popular media has held up a thinner and thinner body ideal for women and a muscular, more buff body image for men. Our culture is obsessed with physical looks and weight, and the importance of each seems to be growing. Nowhere is this more evident than in the media.

Did you know eight-year-old girls talk about dieting?[2] When you ask them why, they'll tell you they are afraid of getting fat! In one study concerning elementary school students and body image, it was found that about 42 percent of first and third graders wished they were thinner.[3] Another survey reported that 40 percent of girls nine and ten years old were trying to lose weight. Where do they get such ideas? One source is through the media they consume.[4]

As long as beauty and success are tied to weight, there will always be a weight-loss market that consumers will drive. Because we can never measure up, we'll buy the products that make us feel like we might be able to at least get in the game. However, psychological fall-out can result from this never ending striving. Children can become depressed and anxious and resort to drastic measures leading to eating disorders.

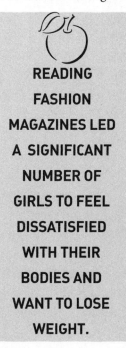

READING FASHION MAGAZINES LED A SIGNIFICANT NUMBER OF GIRLS TO FEEL DISSATISFIED WITH THEIR BODIES AND WANT TO LOSE WEIGHT.

A study reported in the March 1999 issue of *Pediatrics* reinforces what we already fear: young girls are suffering from negative body images and are engaging in unhealthy behaviors as a result.[5] After watching a music video by Britney Spears or viewing a clip from the television show *Friends,* fifth graders told researchers they were dissatisfied with their bodies.[6] *Teen People* magazine conducted a recent survey and found that around a quarter of the teens surveyed felt media pressured them to have perfect bodies.[7] Reading fashion magazines led a significant number of girls to feel dissatisfied with their bodies and to want to lose weight. The images being perpetuated by the media are almost impossible to copy, yet when you ask girls who they want to look like, they'll tell you a TV personality or music star.

FOR MANY COMPANIES, WHAT FATTENS THEIR BOTTOM PROFIT LINE ALSO FATTENS KIDS.

Women and girls aren't the only ones putting up with pressure from media—men and boys are feeling pressure to bulk up and build muscle mass. Little boys play with action figures sporting gigantic muscles and super thin waists. When they compare their own bodies to the toys, it can be disconcerting. With boys, size matters. They want to be big and have muscles.

One reason kids feel so much pressure in terms of how they look has to do with the sheer volume of messages that are sent. Fast-food chains spend more than three billion, yes *billion!* dollars each year on advertising aimed mostly at kids. Their creative strategy is to aggressively market related toys, contests, TV shows, movies, and more in order to capture the attention of kids.[8]

Unfortunately, food is seen as a commodity. For many companies, what fattens their bottom profit line also fattens kids. The money spent on food advertising is second only to the amount spent for the auto industry.[9] Kids influence about 250 billion dollars' worth of consumer spending, which means companies are willing to spend big.[10]

Since advertisements create a desire for the products advertised, and since the target is often children, it isn't surprising that kids want sugary, empty-calorie foods. The ads work! Often the very products parents are trying to avoid—high sugar, high fat, and caffeinated—are being sold. Kids don't have the cognitive capacity to figure out that someone is trying

Food for Thought

The average North American girl will watch 5,000 hours of television, including 80,000 ads, before she starts kindergarten! In the United States, thirty-three commercials will be seen per hour during Saturday morning cartoons.[11]

In terms of body image, one study analyzed only the toy commercials seen during Saturday morning TV and found 50 percent of the commercials aimed at girls talked about physical appearance. Interestingly, none of the boy-related commercials brought up the subject.[12]

to sell them something. Because of their developmental stage, children tend to think that ads are merely information about what to buy and eat.

One of the disturbing trends spotted during Saturday morning kid's programming is the bigger and bigger portion sizes that are being pitched to kids. Sit down and watch television with your children on a Saturday morning, and stick around for the commercials. It's truly amazing. At a time when childhood obesity rates are climbing, ads encourage kids to supersize and overeat. Advertisers target children from a very young age.

Television

Here's a frightening fact: other than sleep, children spend more time watching television than doing any other activity. Think about this! In many homes, television is socializing our children in terms of eating and nutrition. Annually, kids are exposed to thousands of junk food commercials and fast-food options, and during children's peak viewing times, food is the most advertised commodity.[13]

The Kaiser Foundation reports that children see forty thousand ads a year on television, and the content of most of these ads is about candy, snacks, and sodas.[14] In terms of research, we can't say that television viewing causes obesity, but we can determine how much TV the average child is watching. Read these statistics:

- The average American child watches 19 hours and 40 minutes of TV per week. This turns out to be more than a thousand hours per year.[15]

- Two-year-olds watch an average of two hours and five minutes of television per day. The American Pediatrics Association for Children recommends that children two and under watch *zero* hours of TV per day![16]

- In terms of day care settings, 70 percent use TV during the day as part of their program.[17]

How is it that children view so much television?[18]

- The percentage of children ages 8–16 with a TV in their bedrooms is 56 percent.

- The percentage of television-time when children ages 2–7 watch without supervision is 81 percent.

- The percentage of time children age 7 and older watch TV with no parents present is 95 percent.

- The percentage of parents who have no rules about television watching for children ages 8 and up is 61 percent.

- The percentage of parents who would like to limit television watching for their children is 73 percent.

- Only 1 in 12 parents require their children to do homework before watching TV.

And here is one of the saddest statistics I've seen in a long time:

- When 4–6-year-olds were asked if they preferred TV or spending time with their dads, 54 percent preferred watching TV.[19]

If you haven't connected the dots yet, the more children watch TV, the more likely they are to be overweight![20] *There is a connection.* Television is considered a sedentary activity. All you do is sit and watch! It does not promote imagination or socialization since it is a passive activity. Since children are in active developmental stages, their attitudes, beliefs, and ideas about the world, as well as physical and social skills, are taking form and being shaped by the information they view. Sitting passively in front of a screen takes away from time spent on other more active forms of recreation.

Finding a Balance

Maybe you feel you have a good balance when it comes to the number of hours your child plays outside versus time spent watching television. Or maybe you need to limit the time your kids spend watching television. For most of us, the question of how much time should be spent on media is an ongoing battle which is fought daily. When your children do watch television, one way to avoid the constant influence of advertisements is to play videos and fast-forward past all the advertisements. It's a small step, but it reduces the number of food advertisements your child sees in a week, and definitely how much television they watch in general since it cuts out about a third of what would normally be seen.

The American Psychological Association (APA) understands the role television plays in obesity and would like the government to ban unhealthy food commercials from appearing during TV programs for children under nine years of age. Although it is unlikely given the legal issues involved, it speaks volumes that this organization which deals with mental health would take this battle on in order to demonstrate the negative impact of television advertisements on children.

Since your children will be exposed to television food ads unless you throw out your television, a sensible strategy is to teach them to become "media literate." This means you should watch TV with them and talk about what you see. Explain to your children that advertisers want to sell the products and make money. Advertisers do not have their audience's best interests in mind and will sell products that aren't good for those who are listening and watching. Together, discuss which products appearing on ads are healthy (this could be an infrequent discussion) and which ones are unhealthy (a more frequent discussion).

In terms of the impact of media on body image, explain to your child that body features of television stars are often changed or enhanced with props, lighting angles, and computer techniques. For example, freckles and lines can be removed, different body parts from different people can be used in a photo, and body doubles are used in movies to make the actor look more perfect. Computers can generate a thinner look or whatever else is needed. Media often portrays perfect bodies that are either not real or the result of cosmetic surgeries or unhealthy practices like starvation, smoking, and excessive exercise.

Turning the Tide on Television

One national survey found that children who watched four or more hours of television a day had significantly more body fat than those who watched less.[21] Consider the following tips when trying to reign in excessive television viewing:

Take the television out of a child's bedroom. When TV is in the bedroom, you can't monitor what is watched unless you are in the bedroom with the child. And a number of children have the bad habit of watching television while they do their homework. Children also find it tempting to turn on the TV and watch when they should be closing their eyes. This is an easy remedy for taking the guesswork out of monitoring your child's viewing time.

Turn it off during meals. Television viewing during meals isolates people and discourages the art of conversation. Mealtimes are an opportunity to talk with your children about their day and hear their thoughts about life, and vice versa.

Limit its use. Say no to unlimited viewing and set time limits.

What About the Magazines . . . ?

Look around your house to see what magazines are in sight. Are they full of stories about diets, achieving the perfect look, or articles on how to build muscle and achieve that body-building look? Are there pictures and photos of scantily clad women and anorexic-looking models? These images and headlines have the potential to influence your children. Get rid of those magazines which focus on weight and image. They aren't doing you any good either!

Numerous studies that support the idea that too much viewing contributes to overweightness and other negative consequences for your child.

The American Academy of Pediatrics recommends that children should not watch more than one to two hours of television per day, and that children under two should not watch TV at all.

Help your child choose appropriate programs. Use the TV guide or other written program of the viewing schedule and highlight the programs in advance that you find acceptable. Children can then pick from the programs listed for the time limits agreed upon. Give them options but retain veto power.

Be a positive media role model. If your children see you plop down in front of the television night after night, they will learn to do the same. Turn off the TV and engage with your family in some other activity.

No more background noise. Instead of using the television for noise, turn on relaxing music, or teach your children that silence is okay.

Bypass the commercials. One way to limit exposure to commercials is to skip watching commercials entirely. Keep the remote handy and either flip past the commercials or turn the set off.

Watch programs with your children and ask questions. It is helpful to a preschooler to have a parent on hand to answer questions and comment on programs. Ask questions like, "Does a person really act like that or was it make-believe?" Children have difficulty distinguishing reality from fantasy. This goes for commercial-viewing too; talk about what is being sold and whether the products are healthy, or even necessary.

With older kids, watching a program together allows you to view the content. While this is time consuming, it informs you as to the influences your child is allowing. Then, you and your child can discuss the appropriateness of the program. The goal is to promote TV discernment. Do spot checks in which you walk in on TV time unannounced in order to check what your children are watching.

Video Games

The major concerns with video games are the length of time they are played, the content of the games in terms of sexual and violent content, and the impact playing has on children's physical activity. Let's take a short quiz on the facing page and see where your child is.

Your Voice Counts

As an informed adult, you can make a difference through your ability to both write letters and vote. Encourage public policy makers to promote more public service announcements regarding healthy food and activity choices. Television can be used for good purposes like educating and promoting healthy lifestyles. The problem is we need more of these good purposes for watching TV instead of merely trying to entertain ourselves.

When you see offensive ads that are inappropriate for kids, product placement you disagree with, or products that you have strong feelings against, write letters or send emails voicing your opinion. You can write to companies and television networks. Children can also send emails to television networks—most have an email address on their websites.

Quiz

1. Does he play electronic games
    almost every day?   YES   NO

2. Does he play for long periods of time,
    (i.e., three to four hours)?   YES   NO

3. Does he play for excitement and thrills?   YES   NO

4. Does he become restless and irritable
    if he can't play?   YES   NO

5. Does he miss social and school events
    because he would rather play games?   YES   NO

6. Does he avoid conversation because
    he is constantly playing?   YES   NO

7. Does he play when he is supposed
    to be doing homework?   YES   NO

8. Does he play whenever he feels like it,
    with no guidelines?   YES   NO

9. Does he argue or lie about how often
    and long he can play?   YES   NO

10. Does he fail to cooperate when you
    try to cut back on game time?   YES   NO

If you answered yes to even just two or three of these questions, then your child is probably playing too many games. Many children actually prefer electronic games to television viewing.

In a recent study that looked at environmental factors and obesity, video game playing, which is another sedentary activity, was associated with childhood obesity.[22] The good news is, like television, you can set limits on the amount of time video games are played. Again, the purpose is to engage your child in other activities that promote health; by limiting time for video games, you open up time for other physical activity to occur.

In terms of advertising, the number of ads placed in electronic games is rising as a way to offset increasing prices of producing and marketing these games, which means parents need to be vigilant teaching discernment in this venue as well as television. There is also concern about the amount of time electronic games occupy a child's life, especially when you look at game-playing behavior in teens and young adults. Some teens report feelings that they are addicted and have to play video games. Kids can spend hours logging in with multiple players on online games. As a result, they can lose sleep and may not keep up with their schoolwork and other responsibilities.

It appears there may be some truth to the level of addiction felt by some. Studies show that dopamine, a neurotransmitter (chemical) in the brain, gets triggered by playing these games.[23] Dopamine is a chemical that makes you feel pleasure and has been linked to other addictions. We need more studies that evaluate the impact of playing video games on children.

Many experts recommend that the total screen time you allow a child on a given day be limited to one to two hours. *Total* screen time includes television and videos, Internet, computer, and video games. Here are tips to help you manage electronic games:

1. Set a time limit for your child to play ahead of time. Use a kitchen timer and set it to buzz or ring when the time is over. If the timer rings and he refuses to stop, take the game away and give a time-out. You might want to restrict his game use for a period of time until you feel he is ready to try again.

2. Don't let your child bargain extra time by saying, "But I'm in the middle of a game," because they are usually in the middle of a game. Most games have a save button on them and can be stopped and picked up again with no variation in playing. Instruct your child on how to use this feature and tell him to save his game when the time limit is reached.

3. Suggest other activities. If your child is playing video games because

he is bored, engage that child in some other activity. Children need to learn to find other activities which are not screen-oriented to occupy their time.

4. Homework, chores, piano and band practice, and other important tasks should be completed *before* games are played. Work comes before leisure. This lesson must be taught.

5. Take the games out of a child's room. For most kids, having games in their rooms are too tempting.

6. Choose games with your child, play them, and know the ratings. For reasons unrelated to weight, many games contain inappropriate violence and sexual content for kids.

7. When your child does play video games, encourage him to engage in the activity with other children. Add joy sticks and have two or three children play the same game together. I've even seen a family have four joysticks so that four siblings could all play at the same time! At least this way, children are interacting with one another.

MANY EXPERTS RECOMMEND THAT THE TOTAL SCREEN TIME YOU ALLOW A CHILD ON A GIVEN DAY BE LIMITED TO ONE TO TWO HOURS.

The Internet

Most children use the Internet for email, search engines, games, music and homework. As more and more kids go online, advertisers are targeting them. Interactive, animated, and colorful sites are designed to attract children and influence their families' spending. It's a growing business; the hope is that kids will buy into a consumer mentality. And, unlike television, the line between commercials and information is often blurred on the Internet.

Teach your child that advertisers use the Web to push their unhealthy products. Kids should not be clicking on advertising links or giving out personal information. You may even want to build a list of sites that are "advertisement free."

Also be aware that there are some very unhealthy sites on weight loss and dieting. One example is the pro-eating-disorder sites that celebrate dysfunction and provide insider tips on how to maintain dangerously low weights. Pictures of anorexic-looking celebrities are posted. Challenges to keep your weight below 100 pounds are issued. Girls are encouraged to band together and support each other in their desire to stay ill. Ways to hide food and fool friends and relatives are discussed. Former patients brag about noncompliance to eating disorder programs they've attended. Girls are even encouraged to send in pictures of themselves.

I visited several of these sites and felt sick to my stomach. These girls are totally deceived by an enemy who wants them destroyed. Eating disorders are serious and can lead to complicated medical problems, including death. Anyone who celebrates such danger is obviously in need of a renewed mind and healing. And people who desperately try to create community through emotional illness are hurting and need professional help.

Again, the important thing to do is monitor your child's Internet usage. Place a filter on your system, be with your child when he goes online, and teach him how to navigate away from luring ads and unhealthy products and weight solutions. The pop-up ads concerning weight loss are numerous—they have to be sidestepped repeatedly unless you have software that restricts the ads entirely. Talk to your child about these false promises and determine that your family wants to live a healthy life and will make the necessary changes.

Parental Tools for the Internet

If you are unsure about how to go about safeguarding the Internet for your children, check out this website: www.software4parents.com. There is even software available which allows you to see exactly what Web pages were visited and even who was chatted with whom while instant messaging.

A Final Word

The media we have available is so useful when it is used for the right reasons. We cannot take it out of our lives without taking away something extremely valuable. Instead, we need to limit its use. As parents, we have to stay on top of this technology and know what influences are negatively affecting our children. The biggest challenge is one of teaching children balance in terms of how much media is healthy to consume. Parents need to be familiar with media in general and able to teach their children exactly how much time and attention should be given to screen time.

POINTS TO PONDER

1. Overweight kids usually have to cut back on television watching and video game playing. Both are sedentary activities and influence weight gain.

2. Parents should aim for two hours or less of screen media for their children per day.

3. Advertisers target kids in all types of media, even books, and try to influence them to buy unhealthy products that contribute to weight gain.

4. The Internet is another source of child-targeted advertisements. Monitor your child's use and time on the Internet as well as other mediums.

12

When to Seek Professional Help

With short blond hair and a body that looks like it could mow down the defensive line of any opposing team, eleven-year-old Jimmy is 170 pounds and needs to tackle his weight, not people. Since his toddler years, Jimmy consistently stayed in the 99th percentile for weight. When he began kindergarten, he was noticeably one of the largest children in his class. By the end of the third grade, this young boy began to experience physical problems during recess and physical education. He just couldn't keep pace with the other children and instead found himself out of breath and panting just to keep up.

Jimmy's parents were frustrated. After several failed attempts to motivate their son to exercise, they felt like giving up and giving in. "Exercise" had become a dirty word and Jimmy spent most of his day with his Game Boy and video games. In his mind, the risk of teasing and rejection wasn't worth the effort to try and socialize anymore. Jimmy's parents grew more desperate when their pediatrician warned that changes had to be made or Jimmy's health would be compromised.

Furthermore, the teasing and isolation were beginning to take a toll on Jimmy's personality. The once cheery child was becoming more irritable and sneaking food behind his

(Cont'd)

parents' backs. The more his mom and dad tried to structure his eating, the more he rebelled.

The situation felt out of control. Jimmy and his parents needed outside intervention and heard about a Healthy Kids program at a local hospital. The family agreed to give it a try.

Most of you reading this book will be able to make the necessary changes in your family and your child's environment in order to help your child grow into his or her weight. There are times, however, when more help is needed. If that is the case, don't be embarrassed or feel like a failure. Many community hospitals and specialized clinics offer weight-loss programs for children who are significantly overweight or obese. The best candidates for these programs are kids who are in good physical and psychological shape, and who are 30 percent or more overweight.[1] If you are unsure whether seeking professional help is a good alternative for your child, here are some helpful guidelines to consider:

- Like Jimmy's family, you have been trying to make changes for a number of months, but your child is not changing his or her exercise or eating habits. Both you and your child are frustrated because nothing is changing.

- Your health care provider recommends a weight-loss program for your child and your child is 30 percent or more overweight.

- You think eating is meeting a need that you don't quite understand—you believe your child may be eating compulsively. Despite your best efforts to talk with your child about emotional eating, this behavior continues and appears to be out of control.

- You are very worried and unable to stop nagging your child about his eating habits. You know this isn't helping, but you continue to do it out of fear and anxiety.

- Your child is trying to lose weight but doesn't need to do so. She seems preoccupied with food and is fluctuating in her weight. This could be the beginning of the development of an eating disorder. The sooner you seek help, the better your chances are of nipping this problem in the bud and redirecting your child to healthy eating. See the section later in this chapter for signs and symptoms of anorexia, bulimia, compulsive overeating and binge eating.

- Your child seems to be sadder than normal. The sadness seems to stay with her. You notice that she is isolating more in her room, losing interest in activities, and failing subjects in school. She is more irritable, sleeping more or less, having trouble concentrating, making statements about feeling worthless or bad, easily angered, reporting physical pains like stomachaches and headaches that don't seem to have a cause, tired or the opposite—more hyperactive—talking about ending it all or wishing she could disappear. These are signs of childhood depression and must be treated by a physician or mental health professional.

- Your child seems to be lonely and have no close friends. You may want to consider counseling or therapy in order to help your child address this very important aspect of her life.

- You have questions or concerns you've been unable to answer. There is no shame in asking for help when a problem seems to be over your head and everything you are trying isn't moving things forward. Sometimes a third person can be more objective and help you see things differently in order to make new suggestions.

- You feel stuck in your own weight and food obsession and don't feel you can help your child when so much of your time and energy is spent trying to help yourself. I recommend that you purchase a copy of the book *Lose It for Life* co-authored by Stephen Arterburn and myself and begin your own healing journey while helping your child.

Diet Plans Have Some Merit

Even though I have been adamant that you not put your child on a diet, there are times when a doctor-guided weight-loss program should be implemented. Like most things in this life, there are exceptions to the rule. Physicians usually get involved when a child is 30 percent or more overweight. He or she may recommend a professionally staffed children's program in which dieting will not be emphasized but healthy living and eating habits will be developed. These programs usually include:

- *A food diary in which your child records where she eats, type and quantity of food eaten, and who else was present when eating.* This diary is used to figure out eating habits, patterns, and food selection. It is *not* used to calculate calories.

- *A food plan.* A dietitian will work on developing a balanced diet with you and your child. Emphasis will be on eliminating junk food and eating food with high nutritional value.

- *Physical activity.* Professional programs will teach your child ways to be more active. They should provide movement classes and talk to kids about ways to move their bodies more often.

- *Skill building.* If your child eats when he feels upset or bored, or for other emotional reasons, these programs have counselors that will help him develop new ways to cope with negative feelings. For example, he may have to learn to be more assertive or implement a new way to deal with anger when it is felt.

- *Behavioral strategies.* Look for a program that teaches kids lifestyle changes. You want the changes to last and be a part of everyday life.

- *Group support.* Kids learn well in groups, where they benefit from talking to others and learn they aren't alone in this problem. Groups also help with socialization.

- *A counselor or dietitian's advice.* You will probably need help in eliminating foods in your home that are contributing to obesity. These professionals will recommend what to restock your pantry with and teach you more about nutrition. You may need additional help organizing meals and eating at more regular times.

- *Realistic goals.* You and your child must set realistic goals for weight loss. If a child is very obese, the changes that are made should result in a small weight loss each week. Again, weight loss is not the focus, but for those children who are very obese, weight loss will occur when new structure is added to the home and when children eat differently and move more.

I've specialized in the treatment of eating disorders for twenty years and have noticed that the children I treat are now younger and younger. Today, it is not uncommon to have a nine-year-old showing signs of a budding eating disorder. Eating disorders involve a preoccupation with food, weight, and shape that isn't normal. Though they are called "eating disorders," such problems are not just about food. Dieting and weight focus may be an obvious beginning to an eating disorder, but there is much more involved. Otherwise, we would all have eating disorders!

Eating Disorders

Most eating disorders emerge around two critical times in a child's development—the time of puberty and when a young person prepares to leave for home. These are developmental times of stress. As a child's body changes and she is faced with emerging sexuality and pressure to develop her own identity, she may find herself obsessing over food as a way to control feelings that seem out of control. Another time of intense stress is during the time of developmental launching that usually begins in high school and continues as teens move away from home to attend college or enter the job market. This developmental transition requires independence and an increasing self identity.

The Birth of an Eating Disorder

Lauren sat in her room staring at the huge poster of Mary Kate and Ashley Olsen hugging the wall across from her bed. As she stared at the bodies of the two pop culture icons, she felt depressed. How could she ever look like either of those two people? She tried skipping breakfast every day, but she was so hungry by lunchtime that she overate in the school cafeteria. Food was everywhere, yet she was supposed to look like Mary Kate and Ashley. How could she make this happen?

One of the girls in her class suggested she go into the bathroom after lunch and stick her fingers down her throat in order to make herself throw up. If she could make herself vomit, she could eat whatever she wanted at lunch and not worry about getting fat. Lauren tried it once but couldn't bring herself to do it again. It hurt her throat and she hated that gagging feeling. But maybe she would try it again. Her friend Jenna said she did it every day at school and could eat whatever she wanted at lunch and not gain weight.

For the next few weeks, Lauren tried to make herself vomit after lunch. One friend told her that if she ate ice cream and drank milk, vomiting was easier. After a few weeks of practice, she was able to vomit every day. She started to lose weight. One of the teachers noticed and complimented her on her weight loss. Lauren felt so much better as she began to drop the weight. Then she realized she could go to her bathroom after dinner and make herself throw up at home too. If she carefully cleaned up the toilet and sprayed some air freshener, no one would suspect a thing. In fact, her parents seemed to be unaware of any of the changes taking place in Lauren's body because they were so preoccupied with Grandma's cancer treatments.

Lauren's mom seemed very sad and withdrawn as she spent most of her days attending to her mother's needs in the hospital. Lauren wasn't sure what was happening and tried to ask questions about Grandma's health, but no one wanted to talk about it. When she visited the hospital with her mom, Lauren noticed how thin and gaunt Grandma had become. At night, Lauren felt scared that her mom would be so sad she wouldn't be able to care for Lauren anymore if Grandma passed away.

(Cont'd)

In school, another friend told Lauren that she exercised every night in her room. She was able to do one hundred sit-ups and was trying to do them every night. Lauren thought exercise might help her lose more weight and so she decided to try the sit-ups. Doing the sit-ups helped her not think about food and eating, which she liked since it seemed like that was all she thought about anymore. Eventually, Lauren was doing one hundred sit-ups a night and became upset if she couldn't exercise before bed. Some nights when she felt uneasy, she would get up out of bed and do sit-ups to calm down.

Lauren wasn't sleeping well and began to drop even more weight. Now the teacher seemed worried because Lauren looked not only thinner, but also pale and exhausted. But Lauren kept looking at her poster and feeling she was getting closer and closer to the look she thought would make her happy.

Eventually, Lauren's mom noticed the weight drop and took Lauren to the pediatrician for a physical. Lauren had lost 15 percent of her body weight and was still losing weight. She was throwing up two to three times a day and exercising compulsively in her room. The pediatrician told Lauren she was bulimic and needed help. Lauren felt she couldn't stop doing what she was doing—it was almost as though the food and exercise were controlling her. Feeling out of control, Lauren wanted to stop and knew she needed help.

Many factors can influence the development of eating disorders: cultural pressure to be thin and beautiful, gender role expectations and changes, family patterns, personality factors, physiological predispositions, and experience revolving around loss, abuse, and other trauma. Eating disorders are a serious problem and not to be dealt with lightly. Because there is almost always other reasons and emotional issues involved besides food, counseling is recommended, and the sooner the better.

It is important to help girls and boys free themselves from cultural prescriptions of beauty and body image. Kids with eating disorders often try to be perfect; they tend to be compliant and stuff negative feelings away. They often need help setting realistic expectations regarding performance at school. Relationship issues are primary. Conflict is avoided or handled in a poor fashion. Children with eating disorders tend to think in all-or-nothing terms. Life is either all bad or all good—there is no middle ground or balance in thinking or behavior.

Family members are often frightened by the eating behavior because of the seriousness of related medical problems and because the person is misusing food. Children and teens with eating disorders tend to try to take care of family members or other people in their lives while denying their own needs and care. In many cases, fathers are emotionally uninvolved and disconnected with the daughters, unsure how to relate to their daughters' developmental changes and growing independence. Mothers, sensing things are not right, tend to be over- or under-involved with their daughters, unsure how to help them grow and separate emotionally. In general, siblings tend not to be connected as a group.

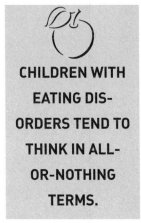

CHILDREN WITH EATING DISORDERS TEND TO THINK IN ALL-OR-NOTHING TERMS.

Typical family patterns include difficulty communicating and directly managing conflict, and also negative emotions. Usually there is marital conflict in which the person with the eating disorder becomes the peacemaker or deflector. In anorexic families, there is usually little emotion expressed. Family conflict is denied while the child tries to compensate by being perfect, and part of this reality is that appearance is very important too. In bulimic families, problems aren't denied; they just aren't resolved. The eating symptoms are an unsuccessful attempt to control and resolve problems and to bring the family together.

Parenting is often done in extreme fashion, such as being overprotective and rigid or else very chaotic. This results in the child feeling guilty, overwhelmed, lonely, and unwilling to developmentally separate from the family and face the challenges of growing up. Eating disorders are a desperate attempt to push away from the family system while staying connected. The conflict is this: the child wants to grow up, but at the same time, she is frightened and feels unprepared to do so. The eating problems keep her family involved by keeping them in a role of caretaker.

The Signs

There is no single event or moment that propels a child into an eating disorder. Multiple issues are involved and develop over time. In general, if your child is developing an eating disorder, you would see these signs:

1. An intense fear of gaining weight

2. A denial of hunger

3. Secretive or deceptive behavior concerning food, like hiding a school lunch or lying about eating a meal

4. An avoidance of food or preoccupation with it

5. Compulsive exercise

6. Cutting food into small pieces and moving it around the plate without eating much

7. Food rituals such as needing to eat the same food out of the same bowl

8. Behavior changes

9. Sleep problems

10. Wearing baggier clothes

Anorexia. This disorder involves an intense fear of gaining weight. Children begin to starve themselves to the point of threatening their lives. Signs of anorexia include weight loss (15 percent or more below an acceptable weight) and refusal to gain weight. Sufferers have a body image disturbance; they do not see themselves clearly and think they are fat even when they are extremely thin. Menstruating females may experience a loss of menses due to the stress the body is experiencing.

Other signs include a preoccupation with weighing food and obsessing over calories, tending to be excessive about exercise, weighing multiple times a day, and discussion of foods as "good" or "bad." Other physical signs include:

- Symptoms related to weight loss (dry skin and hair, cold hands and feet, weakness, constipation, digestive problems, more infections, ketosis, stress fractures, osteoporosis, heart problems, mild anemia, swollen joints)

- Anxiety when eating with others

- Fatigue

- Feelings of worthlessness and hopelessness

- Signs of depression (loss of interest in things, poor concentration, irritability, agitation, restlessness, withdrawal, sleep problems, suicidal thoughts). If your child has several of these signs, see a mental health care provider immediately.

Bulimia. This eating disorder is characterized by binge-purge cycles similar to what is described above. During a binge, large amounts of food are consumed while feeling out of control. Purging follows recurrent episodes of binge eating. Many methods of purging (getting rid of the food) are used. These methods are vomiting, taking laxatives, diuretics, diet pills, exercising excessively, using enemas, fasting, or drinking Ipecac syrup to induce vomiting. Most children won't know about all of these methods of purging, but some will experiment with vomiting after eating a big meal and feeling uncomfortable. As they get older, children usually hear about other ways to get rid of food, whether from other teens or through the media.

Bingeing and purging must occur at least twice a week for a three-month period in order to be clinically diagnosed. Along with the binge-purge cycle, a bulimic child or teen usually obsesses about body weight and shape. She fears being out of control and gaining weight and employs purging to compensate for binges. This explains why many

The Face of Bulimia

Jessica liked to be alone in the house. She didn't have to hide her secret. She would open the refrigerator and it would start. First, she would start with ice cream, then a half-dozen cookies, a liter of Coke, and then leftover pizza and chips. In about ten minutes, Jessica consumed close to 5000 calories and felt sick to her stomach. And she knew her binge would lead to weight gain, which was her biggest fear.

Feeling sick and fat, Jessica ran upstairs and stuck her fingers down her throat. She hung her head over the toilet until she could vomit no more. Then quickly and methodically, Jessica cleaned up the mess and went to sleep on the couch. Jessica's moments of house freedom were really moments of bondage as she struggled in a battle with bulimia.

bulimic sufferers typically keep their weight down. Bingeing and purging is usually secretive and associated with feelings of shame.

Bulimia can bring on the following medical problems:

- Stomach rupture, which is rare but does happen
- Heart failure due to loss of vital minerals such as potassium
- Wearing away of the teeth enamel from acid when vomiting
- Scarring on the backs of hands from having fingers in the mouth to vomit
- Inflamed esophagus
- Swollen cheek glands
- Irregular menstrual periods
- Intestinal problems due to constant irritation of the colon from laxative abuse
- Kidney problems from abuse of diuretics
- Dehydration and electrolyte imbalance

This disorder is related to intense feelings of being out of control. While food is the substance used to numb out emotional pain and difficulty, underlying issues must be faced. Food is often used as a coping mechanism for anger, anxiety, depression, and stress related to multiple areas of a young girl's life. The longer it takes to get help, the more ingrained the habit becomes.

Compulsive and Binge Eating. Another type of compulsive eating is called binge eating. Binge eating is similar to bulimia because the person experiences uncontrolled eating episodes (binges). The difference is that binge eaters don't purge. They eat until they are uncomfortably full. Most binge eaters are obese and struggle with weight fluctuations.

Compulsive overeaters usually overeat due to emotional issues and stress, not because they are hungry. They diet often because of guilt and weight gain and constantly feel out of control when eating. Compulsive eaters tend to be disgusted with their bodies because they are overweight. They may either binge once or twice or overeat throughout the day. The telltale sign of compulsive overeating is usually the fact that the person is overweight or obese.

A Compulsion to Eat

Julie is frustrated with her weight. She has been steadily gaining for months and feels she can't stop bingeing on candy. The more her weight goes up, the more depressed she becomes. Every night she promises herself that she'll be "good." Tomorrow she'll start a diet and get control of her eating. But tomorrow turns out like today—she eats compulsively.

It's hard for Julie to tell the difference between physical hunger and eating out of boredom or stress. She hates feeling this out of control and won't look at her body in the mirror. Julie is a compulsive overeater who doesn't binge eat but instead "grazes" all day on junk food. She picks a little here and a little there until she has grossly overeaten and gained weight.

Where Do Eating Disorders Begin?

Your child's eating patterns may be a predictor of a later problem. For example, we know that picky eaters and children who eat dirt or other substances (a condition called "pica") are at risk for developing eating disorders. Another risk factor is digestive problems in childhood.[2]

In terms of a child's personality, risk factors are low self-esteem, perfectionism, difficulty expressing feelings, people-pleasing behavior, difficulty being assertive, and fear of adulthood. Kids with these other potential characteristics are also at risk:

- Are teased or bullied
- Believe they must meet high expectations of parents
- Go through life-altering experiences such as divorce
- Accumulate multiple, more minor life stresses
- Feel strong peer pressure to conform
- Buy into media images of needing the perfect body
- Feel judged by others because of their appearance

Parents who promote thinness, dieting, and excessive exercise in an attempt to attain ideal bodies are also a significant influence in the development of eating disorders in children. As mentioned before, commenting on your child's weight or shape doesn't help children when it comes to eating disorders. Mothers who comment about their own weight, or the weight of their daughters, negatively influence daughters. Dads who are concerned about thinness influence their daughters' concerns too. For sons, it's the dad's comments about the son's weight that impact the most.

What this all means is that parents need to be very careful not to make negative comments, tease, or ridicule children. If you are a mother with an eating disorder, you need to get professional help now as you are influencing your daughter's eating habits and feelings about her own body. If you are a parent with any kind of untreated psychiatric disorder or significant family problem, get treatment and resolve issues as they may influence children to cope with problems through the unhealthy use of food.

Keep in mind that most children do not typically exhibit all the signs of an eating disorder. Instead, you will notice some of the symptoms as children begin to develop unhealthy eating practices that are precursors to full-blown problems. However, the sooner you recognize a budding problem and begin to address it, the easier it will be to treat it.

Finding the Right Program for You

Currently, there are no weight-loss drugs approved for children. Surgical procedures used on children have not been widely studied and can be very dangerous. With the growing interest in surgical solutions to weight problems, it is recommended that you talk to surgeons on both sides of the issue. Seek out those who do and don't do these surgeries to get their varying perspectives. It's a good idea to get a second opinion regardless when it comes to having your child evaluated for either medical weight-loss programs or other methods of treatment. Here are some important aspects to consider when choosing the right program for you and your child:

1. Look for a program with a variety of health professionals involved. It should include registered dieticians, exercise physiologists, pediatricians or family doctors, and mental health care providers.

2. A medical evaluation should be an initial part of any good program. A physician should review your child's weight, growth, and health before you begin. These should be reviewed during the program on a regular basis as well.

3. A dietitian or nutritionist should provide an individually tailored eating plan for your child based on his food diary and report from his parents.

4. A mental health professional should evaluate your child for any emotional issues or family problems that may be blocking good eating habits.

5. The program should involve your family and not just your child. Children live with their parents, and the changes that are made need to be reinforced at home as well.

6. A good program will be age-sensitive, meaning it will be geared around the capabilities of your child and her developmental needs. A program for a kindergartner should be different than a program for a ten-year-old, particularly in the area of child and parent responsibility.

7. A good program should be able to produce behavioral changes. You shouldn't have to guess if the program is working. Changes should be obvious and observable.

8. A good program will teach your child how to select a variety of foods as well as teaching her what the correct portion sizes should be.

9. Physical activity should be promoted and sedentary activity reduced.

10. Short-term goals that are met should be rewarded in order to motivate and encourage your child to keep making changes. Food and monetary rewards are not recommended.

11. A good program will refer to supports that help maintain the changes. There may be additional underlying emotional issues that may not have been addressed or eating habits that will need continued modification by a qualified professional.

Professional help is available, and I would strongly encourage you to seek it if you see warning signs emerging. I have worked with a number of families with a child on the brink of developing these disorders. Yet with a little help and therapy, things really turned around. There is reason to be hopeful.

POINTS TO PONDER

1. There are definitely times when professional help is needed. It doesn't mean you have failed your children if you need to utilize a weight-loss program.

2. Professional weight-loss programs are designed for obese children who need more supervision and monitoring than parents can give. Criteria for those programs are given.

3. Watch for signs of an eating disorder. Dieting is often an entrée into the problem. While these disorders affect more girls than boys, the percentage for boys is rising.

4. Time is of the essence when treating eating disorders. Don't put off intervention if you see signs. Please seek help.

Epilogue

You Can Do This

In the familiar story of *The Wizard of Oz,* Dorothy desperately seeks an audience with the wizard. She believes that if she can personally speak to him, he will solve both her problem and those of her traveling companions. After a dangerous and arduous trip to Oz, she finally arrives. But then there is a shocking discovery: the wizard, the presumed source of all wisdom and help, is a fake. He's a mousy little guy who sits behind a curtain and pretends to be what he is not—all powerful and all wise. Though he has no real answers, he tries to help Dorothy anyway. Ultimately, his plan fails. Dorothy, now even more distraught, discovers that all this time, she has had the power to go home and didn't know it. With a click of her famous red sparkling shoes, she is transported safely back to Kansas. All is well. End of story.

Sometimes we run around like a bunch of Dorothys . . . we search for wisdom in places it won't be found. Oh, we don't miss a segment of Dr. So and So, or hesitate to write to Dear Whomever for advice. We call in, write in, and email our questions to whomever is the recognized expert voice of the hour. Mind you, there is nothing wrong with asking experts for advice and help. (Otherwise I would not have even written this book!) We benefit from research, people's experiences, and objective experts analyzing a situation. However, we can get so caught up in seeking expertise and knowledge that we forget where our help comes from and who the Author of hope really is.

As you close the pages of this book, I trust you will feel encouraged.

There is much you can do to make a difference in the life of your over-weight child. Your son or daughter doesn't have to struggle with weight for life. Changes can be made. The knowledge you have gained from this book will be very useful, but you need more than knowledge and expertise in order to fully tackle this problem. You need liberal doses of wisdom from the original source, the Bible. According to the book of Proverbs in the Old Testament, wisdom is more precious than rubies; and knowledge is better than gold (8:10–11). A high price is placed on wisdom and understanding because they help us put principles of right living into daily practice. We can never be fully prepared to handle all of life's curve balls, but we can go to the true Source of all wisdom and expect help. When we struggle with any issue, like Dorothy, we need to realize that we already have an answer for the help we need.

Wisdom is different from knowledge. According to Webster, to have knowledge means to "be acquainted with the facts from the study of a certain condition."[1] Reading this book has given you knowledge about weight and children, which is a good thing. Wisdom, however, involves discernment. When the knowledge of what is true is coupled with judg-ment in action, wisdom is at work. For example, you can be knowledge-able about the impact of negative words on a child's self-esteem. You can understand the hurt this presents. But it takes wisdom to respond to the hurt and repair your child's esteem.

God tells us that if we ask anything in His name, He'll do it (John 14:14). And since prayer is our way of communicating with God, it is through prayer we come to God and make our requests known. As parents, ask God to help you make necessary changes and to provide the wisdom needed to parent your overweight child.

Children act as mirrors, reflecting hidden areas of insecurity and fear in parents. Here's an example: I was talking to a friend one day, and she shared how much her daughter's overeating bothered her. She was worried that her daughter was getting fat. One reason this bothered her so much was because she had been an overweight child herself. For years, she endured teasing because of her weight. When I asked her how she resolved the hurt and rejection from her past, she replied, "I haven't. I'm still battling the messages from my mom, the trauma of attending a 'weight camp,' and never feeling good about my body. How do I help my daughter when I don't even know what to do myself? I just feel afraid for her and find myself upset with her a lot."

"That's understandable," I answered, "but it might be best to work on your own weight issues and be healed from past hurts so you don't have to operate in fear and rejection. Then use what you learn to help your daughter. If you work on your issues, you'll help her tremendously. There are people who can help you. God can heal you. You don't have to do this alone. And you don't have to repeat the mistakes your mom made with you. But you've got to gain understanding, receive healing, and ask for wisdom before you can move forward."

Asking for wisdom isn't a difficult thing to do. You simply pray and stay humble. The humble person knows he or she doesn't have all the answers all the time and isn't afraid to admit it. Humble parents understand that their own issues, left unattended and unresolved, often blind them from using good sense with their kids. Yet even when parents do well, things can still go wrong. Therefore, the humble parent spends a great deal of time asking God for His wisdom, reading His life-giving principles found in the Word, and listening for His voice. There is recognition that moving in one's own strength leads to defeat. We need to pray for God's will to be done, be obedient to His Word, listen for His voice, and move according to His plan.

Nothing can match what God can give you. He is perfect, righteous, sovereign, holy, merciful, and wise in all things. To fear God with a sacred awe of who He is and to recognize His omnipotence, majesty, and goodness brings us to a place of submission. We need Him. To operate apart from the wisdom of God brings anxiety. We need Him in all we do, especially when parenting our children in today's world. Instead of becoming desperate for your children to lose weight, be desperate to know God more each day. Be a glutton for Him!

Thankfully, there is grace for parenting! As we acknowledge our faults and mistakes, God's grace is sufficient and covers over a multitude of sins. Don't stress about one comment or parenting mistake—weight problems and eating disorders are the result of patterns. Instead, confess the problem and move on.

Come and Dine

God cares about the weight struggles you face. Yet He has so much more for you and your children. As you provide nutritious food, become more physically active, and learn to adopt a healthier lifestyle, God wants you to feast regularly on His spiritual food. This food will sustain and nurture your souls and spirits. The invitation has been given. The table has been set. Jesus calls us to come with a hearty appetite.

In John 6, Jesus instructs us not to waste our energy striving for perishable food. He knows that the food of this earth will never satisfy the deeper longing He has placed in each of us for Him. Jesus refers to himself as the Bread of Life, the Bread that came down from heaven and gives life to this world. Anyone who eats this Bread will not be hungry and will live eternally with God.

Jesus also calls Himself the Living Water. If we believe in Him and drink of His spirit, we will never thirst again. What incredible promises—to never be hungry or thirsty again. As we desire more of Him and open our mouths, He feeds us and nourishes our spirits. This is what sustains us and gives us hope.

As I was reading the words of Jesus recorded in the Gospel of John, I remembered an old hymn I used to sing as a child:

"Come and Dine"[2]

Jesus has a table spread

Where the saints of God are fed

He invited His chosen people

Come and dine.

With His manna, He doeth feed

And supplies our every need

O 'tis sweet to sup with Jesus all the time.

Come and dine the master's calling

Come and dine.

You may feast at Jesus' table all the time.

He who fed the multitudes,

Turned the water into wine.

To the hungry calleth now

Come and dine.

Soon the Lamb will take His bride

To be ever at His side

All the hosts of heaven

Will assembled be.

Oh twill be a glorious sight

All the saints in spotless white

And with Jesus they will feast eternally.

This song is an invitation to come and dine with the One who created us and longs to give us exactly what we need. Unless we are willing to sit down and experience this spiritual food, there will always be a void in our lives which we will attempt to fill with the unhealthy use of food and other substances. Jesus patiently waits for us to come and is delighted when we want more of Him.

Will you "taste and see that the Lord is good"? Will you offer your children spiritual food that will satisfy their souls and bring them to a place of peace and contentment in a world that has neither? The table is set. The feast is ready, and like Dorothy, we already have what we need. What hope we have in Christ! Be encouraged.

I keep asking that the God of our Lord Jesus Christ, the glorious Father, may give you the Spirit of wisdom and revelation, so that you may know him better. I pray also that the eyes of your heart may be enlightened in order that you may know the hope to which he has called you, the riches of his glorious inheritance in the saints, and his incomparably great power for us who believe. That power is like the working of his mighty strength.

EPHESIANS 1:17–19

Growth Chart for Boys, Age 0–36 Months

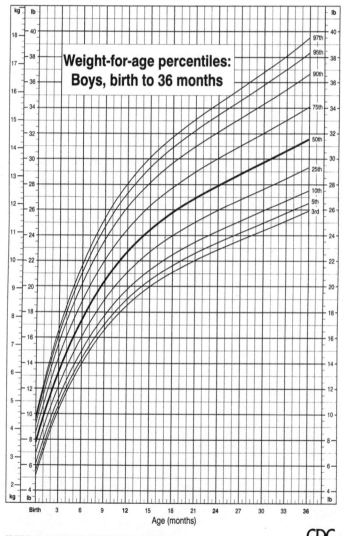

Weight-for-age percentiles: Boys, birth to 36 months

SOURCE: Developed by the National Center for Health Statistics in collaboration with the National Center for Chronic Disease Prevention and Health Promotion (2000).

Figure 1. Weight-for-age percentiles, boys, birth to 36 months, CDC growth charts: United States

Growth Chart for Girls, Age 0–36 Months

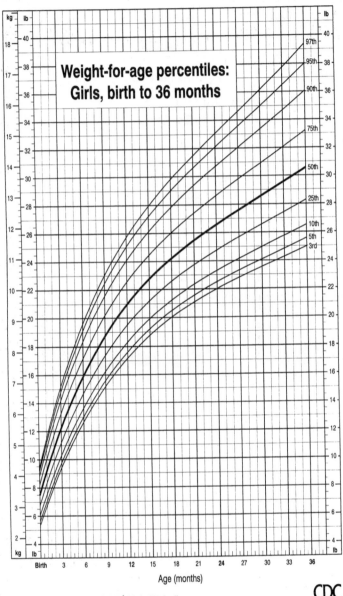

Figure 2. Weight-for-age percentiles, girls, birth to 36 months, CDC growth charts: United States

Growth Chart for Boys, Ages 2–20 Years

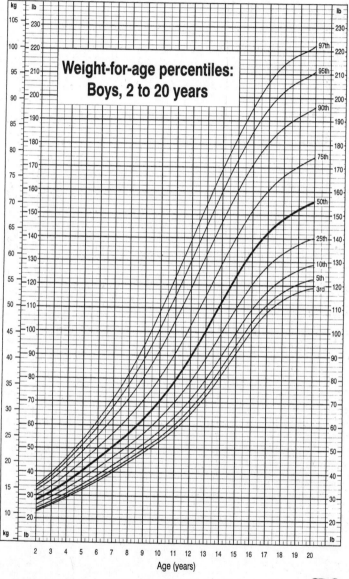

Weight-for-age percentiles:
Boys, 2 to 20 years

SOURCE: Developed by the National Center for Health Statistics in collaboration with
the National Center for Chronic Disease Prevention and Health Promotion (2000).

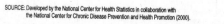

Figure 9. Weight-for-age percentiles, boys, 2 to 20 years, CDC growth charts: United States

Growth Chart for Girls, Age 2–20 Years

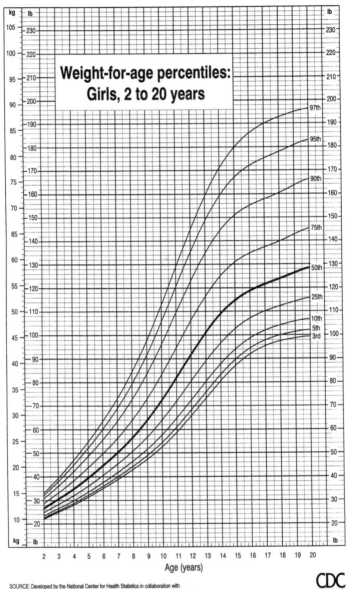

SOURCE: Developed by the National Center for Health Statistics in collaboration with
the National Center for Chronic Disease Prevention and Health Promotion (2000).

Figure 10. Weight-for-age percentiles, girls, 2 to 20 years, CDC growth charts: United States

Appendix B: BMI Charts

BMI for Boys

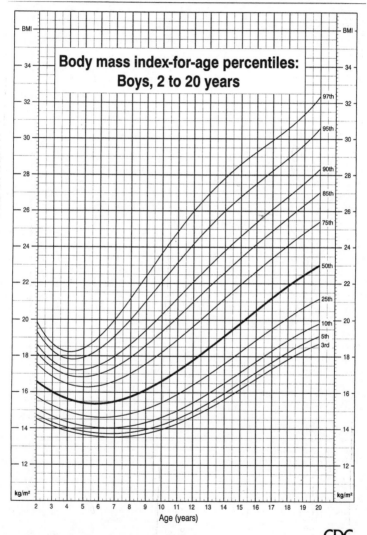

Body mass index-for-age percentiles:
Boys, 2 to 20 years

SOURCE: Developed by the National Center for Health Statistics in collaboration with
the National Center for Chronic Disease Prevention and Health Promotion (2000).

CDC

Figure 15. Body mass index-for-age percentiles, boys, 2 to 20 years, CDC growth charts: United States

BMI for Girls

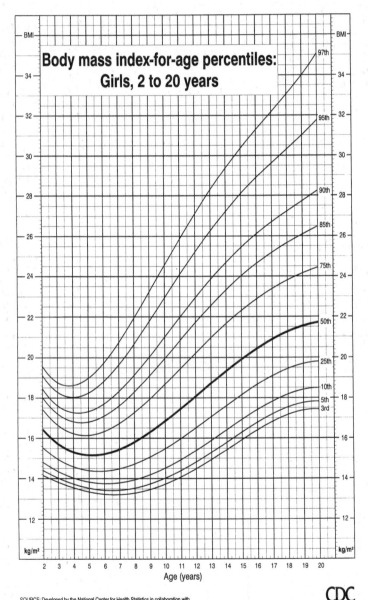

Figure 16. Body mass index-for-age percentiles, girls, 2 to 20 years, CDC growth charts: United States

Appendix C: Inspirational Scriptures

Genesis 1:27

So God created man in his own image, in the image of God he created him; male and female he created them.

Psalm 139:13–14

For you created my inmost being; you knit me together in my mother's womb. I praise you because I am fearfully and wonderfully made; your works are wonderful, I know that full well.

Ephesians 2:10

For we are God's workmanship, created in Christ Jesus to do good works, which God prepared in advance for us to do.

1 Corinthians 3:16

Don't you know that you yourselves are God's temple and that God's Spirit lives in you?

1 Samuel 16:7

But the LORD said to Samuel, "Do not consider his appearance or his height, for I have rejected him. The LORD does not look at the things man looks at. Man looks at the outward appearance, but the LORD looks at the heart."

1 Peter 3: 3–4

Your beauty should not come from outward adornment, such as braided hair and the wearing of gold jewelry and fine clothes. Instead, it should be that of your inner self, the unfading beauty of a gentle and quiet spirit, which is of great worth in God's sight.

Romans 12:1

Therefore, I urge you, brothers, in view of God's mercy, to offer your bodies as living sacrifices, holy and pleasing to God—this is your spiritual act of worship.

Ephesians 1:3–6

Praise be to the God and Father of our Lord Jesus Christ, who has blessed us in the heavenly realms with every spiritual blessing in Christ. For he chose us in him before the creation of the world to be holy and blameless in his sight. In love he predestined us to be adopted as his sons through Jesus Christ, in accordance with his pleasure and will—to the praise of his glorious grace, which he has freely given us in the One he loves.

Jeremiah 29:11

"For I know the plans I have for you," declares the LORD, "plans to prosper you and not to harm you, plans to give you hope and a future."

Endnotes

Chapter 1: Is My Child Overweight?

1. Reinberg, S., "Many Parents Are Blind to Their Kids' Weight Problems," Health Day (June 4, 2004). Retrieved online July 14, 2004, from http://pediatrics.about.com/b/a/015764.htm

2 Growth charts for boys and girls. Retrieved online November 13, 2004, from http://pediatrics.about.com/cs/growthcharts2/l/bl_growthcharts.htm
Charts published May 30, 2000 (modified October 16, 2000). Developed by the National Center for Health Statistics in collaboration with the National Center for Chronic Diseases and Prevention and Health Promotion (2000). http://www.cdc.gov/growthcharts

3. Reinberg, S., "Many Parents Are Blind to Their Kids' Weight Problems," Health Day (June 4, 2004). Retrieved online July 14, 2004, from http://pediatrics.about.com/b/a/015764.htm

4. National Center for Chronic Disease prevention and health promotion. "BMI for Children and Teens," retrieved online August 10, 2004, from http://www.cdc.gov/nccdphp/dnpa/bmi/bmi-for-age.htm

5. Growth charts for boys and girls. Retrieved online November 13, 2004, from http://pediatrics.about.com/cs/growthcharts2/l/bl_growthcharts.htm
Charts published May 30, 2000 (modified October 16, 2000). Developed by the National Center for Health Statistics in collaboration with the National Center for Chronic Diseases and Prevention and Health Promotion (2000). http://www.cdc.gov/growthcharts

6. "Three-year-old Dies from Obesity," BBC News. Retrieved online August 31, 2004, from http://news.bbc.co.uk/1/hi/health/3752597.stm

7. O'Neill, Brendon, "Choking on the Facts" (June 7, 2004). Retrieved online September 2, 2004, from http://www.spiked-online.com/Printable/0000000CA568.htm

8. Hellmich, N. (June 4, 2004). "Child Obesity Worse than Thought," *USA Today.* Retrieved online at http://pediatrics.about.com/b/a/015764.htm

9. Taken from Center for Nutrition Policy and Promotion, U.S. Department of Agriculture. Symposium proceedings from October 27, 1998, on Childhood Obesity: Causes and prevention. Retrieved online from www.usda.gov.cnpp/Seminars/obesity.PDF

10. Mundell, E.J., "Report Gives Mixed Grades on Kids' Health," (March 24, 2004). Retrieved online July 14, 2004, from http://www.keepmedia.com/ShowItemDetails.do?item_404399&oliID=42&bemID=hizeBFIIjLh7mm2B7n5Mwaa185

11. Centers for Disease Control (2000). "Physical Activity and Youth." Available online at www.cdc.gov/kidsmedia/background.htm (visited 10/11/01).

12. Facts taken from American Obesity Association. AOA Fact Sheet. Obesity in Youth. Retrieved online September 3, 2004, from http://www.obesity.org/subs/fastfacts/obesity_youth.shtml

13. "The Problems of Childhood Obesity. Retrieved online September 7, 2004, from http://www.bupa.co.uk/health_information/html/healthy_living/children/obesity/obesity_problems.html#2

14. Ibid.

15. "Obese Kids More Likely to Have Bowel Problems. Reuters Health Information, taken from *The Journal of Pediatrics,* August 2004. Retrieved online September 3, 2004, from http://www.nlm.nih.gov/medlineplus/news/fullstory_19890.html

16. Richardson, M., "Current Perspectives in Polycystic Ovary Syndrome," *American Family Physician* (August 15, 2003). Retrieved online October 30, 2004, from http://www.aafp.org/afp/20030815/697.html

17. "Overweight: a Weight Reduction Program." Retrieved online July 29, 2004, from http://www.med.umich.edu/libr/pa/pa bwghtred hhg.htm

18. Stacey, M. "Stop Me Before I Eat More!" *O Magazine* (August 2004).

19. Jaret, P., "Breaking the Urge to Eat" *Reader's Digest* (July 2004).

Chapter 2: Let's Talk About It

1. "Success," Merriam-Webster's Colelgiate Dictionary, Springfield, Massachusetts, 2003.

2. Rimm, S., "Rescuing the Emotional Lives of Overweight Children." Retrieved online July 29, 2004, from http://www.sylviarimm.com/RTELOOCart.htm

Chapter 3: Not a Lifelong Battle

1. Cafaro, T. & Bernstein, S., "Children and Weight Management Issues," (July 1, 2004). Retrieved online August 19, 2004, from http://www.medicalmoment.org/_content/signs/jul04/240368.asp

Chapter 4: The Do's and Don'ts of Eating Habits

1. "Preventing Childhood Obesity," (November 2003). Retrieved online July 14, 2004, from http://www.health.harvard.edu/fhg/updates/update1103d.shtml

2. "Study: Toddlers Have Bad Eating Habits," *USA Today,* Posted October 26, 2003. Retrieved online August 31, 2004, from http://www.usatoday.com/news/health/2003-10-26-toddler-eating_x.htm
J Am Diet Assoc. 2004, Jan;104 (1 Suppl 1):s8-13.

3. Zablocki, Elaine, "Variety Is the Spice of Life-for Babies, Too!" WebMD Medical News. (June 19, 2000). Retrieved online January 5, 2005 from http://my.webmd.com/content/article/16/1728_81734.htm

4. Credit for the Food Pyramid for Children goes to the U.S. Department of Agriculture. Information retrieved online on December 23, 2004, from http://www.usda.gov/cnpp/KidsPyra/

5. Mayo Foundation for Medical Education and Research, March 2, 2004. "Sensible Approaches to Children's Weight Problems." Retrieved online on August 15, 2004, from http://www.cnn.com/HEALTH/library/FL/00057.html

6. Obesity Health Warnings. Retrieved online July 20, 2004, from http://www.annecollins.com/obesity/health-warning.htm

7. "Ban Trans Fat." Retrieved online September 13, 2004, from http://www.bantransfats.com/

8. Severson, K., (May 12, 2003). Lawsuit seeks to ban sale of Oreos(tm) to children in California. Nabisco taken to task over trans fat's effects. *The San Francisco Chronicle.* Retrieved online September 13, 2004, from http://sfgate.com/cgi-bin/article.cgi?f=/c/a/2003/05/12/OREO.TMP

9. "Fiber and Children's Diets," AHA Recommendations. Retrieved online September 13, 2004, from http://www.americanheart.org/presenter.jhtml?identifier=4608

10. Spake, A. and Marcus, M., "A Fat Nation," *US News and World Report,* special edition, (August 19, 2002), 40-47.

11. Gilbert, P., "Introduction to Salt and Children," Consensus Action on Salt and Health (CASH). Retrieved online September 13, 2004, from http://www.hyp.ac.uk/cash/children_intro.htm

12. Calcium. kidskeephealthy.com. Retrieved online September 12, 2004, from http://www.keep-kidshealthy.com/nutrition/calcium.html

13. Spake, A. and Marcus, M., "A Fat Nation," *US News and World Report,* special edition, (August 19, 2002), 40-47.

14. "Weight Loss Tips," keepkidshealthy.com. Retrieved online November 12, 2004, from http://www.keepkidshealthy.com/nutrition/weight_loss_for_kids.html

15. Doherty, W., "Overscheduled Kids, Underconnected Families: the research evidence," (2000). http://puttingfamiliesfirst.info/html/research.htlm

16. Gillman, M.W., Rifas-Shiman, S.L., Frazier, A.L., Rockette, H.R.H., Camargo, C.A., Field, A.E., Berkey, C.S., & Colditz, G.A. "Family Dinners and Diet Quality Among Older Children and Adolescents," Archives of *Family Medicine,* (2000). 9,235-240. A questionnaire using 24- hour recall that was mailed to children of participants in the ongoing Nurses Health Study II. Retrieved online October 6, 2004, from http://216.239.41.104/search?q=cache:H5jg_Q0v74J:edprojects.che.umn.edu/take-back/downloads/research.pdf+overscheduled+kids+and+underconnected+families&hl=en

17. Sandra L. Hofferth, "Changes in American Children's Time,"1981-1997." University of Michigan's Institute for Social Research, Center Survey, January, 1999. National probability samples of American families with children ages 3-12, using time diary data from 1981 and 1997. Findings on how time use is associated with children's well-being are reported in Hofferth, S. L., "How American

Children Spend Their Time," *Journal of Marriage and the Family,* (2001).63, 295-308. Retrieved online October 4, 2004, from http://216.239.41.104/search?q=cache:H5jg_Q0-v74J:edprojects.che.umn.edu/takeback/downloads/research.pdf+overscheduled+kids+and+undercon-nected+families&hl=en

18. Robert Putnam, *Bowling Alone: The Collapse and Revival of American Community.* New York: Simon and Schuster, 2000. Putnam reports on the decline in dinners and vacations, using yearly polls of national probability samples of married couple households since the mid-1970s. The dinner question repeated yearly Retrieved online October 4, 2004, from http://216.239.41.104/search?q =cache:H5jg_Q074J:edprojects.che.umn.edu/takeback/downloads/research.pdf+overscheduled+kids +and+underconnected+families&hl=en asked whether "our whole family usually eats dinner together." The percent of married respondents answering "definitely" declined from about 50 percent to 34 percent from 1977-1999. Retrieved online October 6, 2004, from http://216.239.41.104/ search?q=cache:H5jg_Q0v74J:edprojects.che.umn.edu/takeback/downloads/research.pdf+oversched-uled+kids+and+underconnected+families&hl=en

Chapter 5: Eat to Grow...Grow to Eat?

1. Burghart, T., "Weight of Children, Mother Linked, Study Says," *The Virginian-Pilot* (July 6, 2004).
2. Smith, I.V. "Understanding and Preventing Childhood Obesity." Retrieved online July 7, 2004, from http://www.childcare-ppin.com/ezine/health102.htm
3. "Infant Weight Gain Could Be Linked to Later Obesity," *Daily University Science News,* (February 4, 2002). Retrieved online 8/17/04 from http://unisci.com/stories/20021 /0204023.htm
4. "Breastfed Babies Less Likely to Be Overweight Children," *Daily University Science News,* (May 16, 2001). Retrieved online 8/17/04 from http:// http://unisci.com/stories/20012/0516012.htm
5. AskDr.Sears.com. "How much weight should I expect my breastfeeding baby to gain?" Retrieved online August 17, 2004, from http://www.askdrsears.com/html/2/t023600.asp
6. Chart information taken from *Complete Book of Baby & Child Care.* Focus on the Family, Paul C. Reisser, author. Published by Tyndale, 1997.
7. AskDr.Sears.com. "How much weight should I expect my breastfeeding baby to gain?" Retrieved online August 17, 2004, from http://www.askdrsears.com/html/2/t023600.asp
8. Kolp-Jurss, B., "Picky Eaters Need Structure, Medical Moment, (July 1, 2004). Retrieved online August 19, 2004, from http://www.medicalmoment.org_content/helpyourself/jul04/240369.asp
9. Gilbert, S., iVillage. "Guidelines for Toddlers." Retrieved online 8/17/04 from http://www.parentsplace.com/expert/nutritionist/qas/0, 205647_105322,00.html
10. Three-year-olds. Retrieved online August 31, 2004, from http://www.canadianparents.com /preschool/ss_threeyolds.htm
11. Four-year-olds. Retrieved August 31, 2004, online from http://www.canadianparents.com/ preschool/ss_fouryolds.htm
12. Kolp-Jurss, B., "Picky Eaters Need Structure, Medical Moment, (July 1, 2004). Retrieved online August 19, 2004, from http://www.medicalmoment.org_content/helpyourself/jul04/240369.asp
13. *USA Today* (February 12, 2001). Retrieved online from usatoday.com/news/health/2001-01-12-early-puberty.htm
14. Ibid.

Chapter 6: Let's Move!

1. Kimm, S., Glynn. N., Kriska, A., Barton., B., Kronsberg, S., Daniels, S., Crawford, P., Sabry, Z. & K.Lui, "Decline in Physical Activity in Black Girls and White Girls During Adolescence," *New England Journal of Medicine* (September, 2002). 347 (10), 709-715.
2. Exercise (physical activity for children). Retrieved online September 29, 2004, from http://www.americanheart.org/presenter.jhtml?identifier=4596
3. Parr, R. "Exercise for overweight kids," *The Physician and Sports Medicine,* Vol. 6, No. 6, June 1998. Retrieved online November 12, 2004, from http://www.physsportsmed.com /issues/1998/06jun/kids.htm
4. "Raising an Active Child: Ideas for Parents." Mayo Clinic Staff. Retrieved online September 29, 2004, from http://www.mayoclinic.com/invoke.cfm?id=FL00030

5. KidsHealth for Parents. "The Power of Play." Retrieved online November 4, 2004, from http://www.kidshealth.org/parent/growth/learning/power_play.html

6. Permission to list web site granted by Geof Nieboer, Webmaster, www.gameskidsplay.net

Chapter 8: Emotional Feeding Equals Overweight Kids

1. Silverman, W.K., La Greca, A.M., & Wasserstein, S., "What Do Children Worry About?: Worries and Their Relationship to Anxiety," *Child Development,* 66, (1995). 671–686.

2. Henker, B., Whalen, C. K. & O'Neil, R., "Worldly and Workaday Worries: Contemporary Concerns of Children and Young Adolescents," *Journal of Abnormal Child Psychology,* 23, (1995). 685–702.

3. Statistics quoted from the National Child Abuse and Neglect Data System. Reorted online by Matthew Neff, May 1, 2003, HHS releases 2001 national statistics on child abuse and neglect. Newsletter, Brief article from http://www.findarticles.com/p/articles/mi_m3225/is_9_67/ai_102223737

4. US Census Bureau of Household and Family Statistics, 2000.

5. *State of America's Children Yearbook 2000,* Children's Defense Fund.

6. Child stats.gov America's children 2000. Retrieved online October 5, 2004, from http://www.childstats.gov/ac2000/highlight.asp

7. Ibid.

8. The National Commission on Children.

9. Stepfamily Association of America.

10. Strauss, Murray A, Gelles, Richard J., and Smith, Christine *Physical Violence in American Families; Risk Factors and Adaptations to Violence in 8,145 Families.* New Brunswick: Transaction Publishers, 1990.

11. Carlson, Bonnie E., "Children's Observations of Interpersonal Violence," (1984). 147-167 in A.R. Roberts (Ed.) *Battered Women and Their Families* (pp. 147–167). NY: Springer. Straus, M.A. (1992). "Children as Witnesses to Marital Violence: a Risk Factor for Lifelong Problems among a Nationally Representative Sample of American Men and Women. *Report of the Twenty-Third Ross Roundtable.* Columbus, OH: Ross Laboratories.

12. National Statistics: Snapshots of Work and Family in America. Retrieved online from http://www.pbs.org/workfamily/discussion_snapshots.html

13. Ibid.

14. Ibid.

15. Poll conducted in 2002 on a nationally representative sample of 746 children, ages 9-14, for the Center for the New American Dream, Takoma Park, Maryland. Retrieved online October 4, 2004, from http://216.239.41.104/search?q=cache:H5jg_Q0v74J:edprojects.che.umn.edu/takeback/downloads/research.pdf+overscheduled+kids+and+underconnected+families&hl=en

16. Global Strategy Group, Inc., "Talking with Teens: The YMCA Parent and Teen Survey." Final Report, April, 2000. National probability sample of teens who were asked to list their chief concerns. Teens of all ages listed not enough time with their parents as the top concern. Retrieved online October 4, 2004, from http://216.239.41.104/search?q= cache:H5jg_Q0v74J:edprojects.che.umn.edu/takeback/downloads/research.pdf+overscheduled+kids+and+underconnected+families&hl=en

17. Results summarized from http://216.239.41.104/search?q=cache:H5jg_Q0v74J:edprojects.che.umn.edu/takeback/downloads/research.pdf+overscheduled+kids+and+underconnected+families&hl=en Retrieved online October 6, 2004.

18. Picard, Andrew, Public Health Reporter, "Stress Linked to Obesity in School-age Children." Retrieved online October 6, 2005 from http://www.evalu8.org/staticpage?page=review&siteid=3472 (Referenced the August issue of the journal *Health Psychology*).

19. Gunnar, M. R., Sebanc, A., Tout, K., Donzella, B. & van Dulman, M., "Temperament, Peer Relationships, and Cortisol Activity in Preschoolers," *Developmental Psychobiology,* 2003).

20. List copied from website http://www.acf.dhhs.gov/healthymarriage/benefits/index.html from the US Department of Health and Human Services, Administration for Children and Families. The Healthy Marriage Initiative, Wade Horn, PhD , Assistant Secretary. Updated May 24, 2004. Retrieved online October 6, 2004.

21. Reinberg, Steve, "Behavior Problems Feed Childhood Obesity" (November 3, 2003). Retrieved online July 14, 2004, from http://pediatrics.about.com/b/a015764.htm

Chapter 9: Sticks and Stones...Words and Hurts

1. Gardner, A., "Weight Teasing an Emotional Crisis for Kids," (August 11, 2003). Retrieved online July 14, 2004, from http://www.pediatrics.about.com/b/a/015764.htm

2. Mulrine, A., "Once Bullied, now Bullies—with Guns. *US News and World Report,* May 3, 1999, 24.

Chapter 10: Schools Do Play a Role

1. Centers for Disease Control and Prevention, School Health Policies and Programs Study, 2000. Fact sheet on "Food Service." Retrieved online October 14, 2004, from http://www.cdc.gov.nccdphp/dash/shpps/factsheets/fs01_foods_sold_outside_schoolhtm

2. Spake, A. and Marcus, M., "A Fat Nation," *US News and World Report,* special edition, (August 19, 2002), 44-51.

3. Information retrieved online October 14, 2004, from http://www.pta.org/aboutpta/sponsors.asp

4. Ibid.

5. School and school age children. Action Alliance for children. Retrieved online October 16, 2004, from http://www.4children.org/schools.htm

6. "Three Parents Who Made a Difference at Their Schools." Retrieved online October 16, 2004, from http://www.greatschools.net/cgi-bin/showarticle/TX/295/improve

7. Channel One overview. Retrieved online October 12, 2004, from http://www.commercialalert.org/index.php/category_id/2/subcategory_id/32/article_id/120

8. Ibid.

9. "Are schools for sale to advertisers?" April 19, 2000. EagleForum.org Phyllis Sschlafly. Retrieved online October 12, 2004, from http://www.eagleforum.org/column/2000/apr00/00-04-19.html

10. Zoll, M. (April 5, 2000). Psychologist challenge ethics of marketing to children. Mediachallenge.org Retrieved online October 12, 2004, from http://www.mediachannel.org/originals/kidsell.shtml

11. Spake, A. and Marcus, M., "A Fat Nation," *US News and World Report,* special edition, (August 19, 2002), 44-51.

12. Commerical Alert. Retrieved online October 28, 2004, from http://www.commercialalert.org/index.php/category_id/1/subcategory_id/69/article_id/169

Chapter 11: Media's Part in the Equation

1. "Stop Commercial Exploitation of Children: Facts About the Effects of Advertising and Marketing on Children." Retrieved-online July 14, 2004, from http://www.commercial exploitation.com/article/congressional_briefing_facts. htm

2. Panahi, H., "Mirror, Mirror: Fostering a Positive Body Image in Your Child," (September 24, 2004). Retrieved online October 16, 2004, from http://www2.townonline.com/parentsandkids/news/view.bg?articleid=88437&format=

3. Ibid.

4. *USA Today,* (August 12, 1996), 1D.

5. Field, A. Cheung, L. Wolf, A. Herzog, D. Gortmaker, S. and Colditz, G., "Exposure to the Mass Media and Weight Concerns Among Girls," *Pediatrics,* vol. 103 No. 3 (March 1999), 36.

6. Mundell, EJ. "Sitcoms, Videos Make Even Fifth-Graders Feel Fat," (August 26, 2002). Reuters Health accessed at: http://story.news.yahoo.com/news?tmpl=story2&cid=594&ncid= 594&e=2&u=/nm/20020826/hl_nm/obesity_television_dc_1 (last visited 9/16/02)

7. "Body image and advertising." Retrieved online October 16, 2004, from http://www.mediascope.org/pubs/ibriefs/bia.htm

8. Special issues for young children. Developmental concerns. Retrieved online October 27, 2004, from http://www.mediaawareness.ca/english/parents/marketing/issues_kids_marketing.cfm

9. Lappe, F. & Lappe, A., "Obesity? It's Been Programmed Into our Food," *The Virginian-Pilot* (August 7, 2004).

10. The Television Project (2003). Basic data about television watching Retrieved online July 14, 2004, from http://www.tvp.org/Handouts percent20pages/basic_data_txt.html

11. "Media and girls." Retrieved online October 16, 2004, from http://www.media awareness.ca/english/issues/stereotyping/women_and_girls/women_girls.cfm

12. Thompson, T. and Zerbinos, E., "Television Cartoons: Do Children Notice It's a Boy's World?" *Sex Roles: A Journal of Research,* 37, (1997), 415–433.

13. Coon, K. & Tucker, K., "Television and Children's Consumption Matter: a Review of the Literature. *Minerva Pediatrics,* 54 (5), (October 2002), 423–436.

14. Lappe, F. & Lappe, A., "Obesity? It's Been Programmed Into our Food," *The Virginian-Pilot* (August 7, 2004).

15. Neilson Media Research, "2000 Report on Television": 14.

16. Facts and figures about our TV habits. Retrieved online October 5, 2004, from www.tvturnoff.org/images/facts&figs/factsheet/Facts percent20and percent20Figures.pdf

17. Ibid.

18. Ibid.

19. Ibid.

20. Television and obesity. Retrieved online July 14, 2004, from http://www.commercialalert.org/index.php/category id/5/subcategory id/72/article id/236

21. Andersen, R. E., Crespo, C.J., Bartlett, S. J., Cheskin, L. J., Pratt, M., "Relationship of Physical Activity and Television Watching with Body Weight and Level of Fatness Among Children," *Journal of the American Medical Association,* (March 25, 1998), 279, 938-942.

22. "Video Games and Obesity, Best Evidence Yet," (June 30, 2004). Retrieved online October 28, 2004, from http://www.healthcentral.com/drdean/ eanfulltexttopics.cfm?ID=60891&storytype=DeanTopics

23. Ingram, J. (June 12, 1998). EXN.ca Discovery Channel. "Positron Emission Tomography; Retrieved online November 2, 2004, from http://exn.ca/Stories/1998/06/12/59.asp

Chapter 12: When to Seek Professional Help

1. "What about a formal weight loss program?" American Academy of Pediatrics. Medical library. Retrieved online October 23, 2004, from http://www.medem.com/MedLB/article_detaillb.cfm?article_ID=ZZZB92U8W7C&sub_cat=382

2. Emily Majors, "Children and Eating Disorders: a Review of the Literature." Retrieved online October 23, 2004, from http://www.vanderbilt.edu/AnS/psychology/health_psychology/childrenandED.html

Epilogue: You Can Do This

1. Webster's encyclopedia unabridged dictionary of the English language. (1989). New York/Avenel, New   Jersey: Gramercy Books.

2. 100 inspirational gospel favorites. (1977). "Come and Dine"; words by C.B. Widmeyer, music by S.H. Bolton. Compiled by Don Marsh and W. Elmo Mercer. John T. Benson Company.